The Chronicles Of a Critical Care Nurse

By Pamela Karakusis BSN, RN, CCRN, CNC

For information regarding permission, please write to:

Chroniclesofacriticalcarenurse@gmail.com

ISBN-978-0-578-65319-8

Author: Pamela Karakusis

Illustrator: Pamela Karakusis

Editor: Katrina Loving

This book is published by Pamela Karakusis

through KDP Select,

a subsidiary of Amazon.com, Inc.

Printed by Kindle Direct Publishing

Published in the United States of America.

To purchase more copies directly, please visit:

www.amazon.com

To the hummingbird in my life,

Je t’aime!

Flamme Jumelle!

Thank you

To Meg Sakala,

for being my mentor and friend in life.

Your passion for people and for critical care has always inspired me.

My successes in this profession are because of your guidance and support.

To Sue Buszkiewic,

for believing in me before I believed in myself.

I wouldn't be where I am today without you.

To Delinda Romero Fatianow,

for giving me a safe place to express myself.

Your restaurant is part of my creative energy and also my safe haven.

I'm fortunate to call you my friend!

Thank You

To Kristina Alvarez and Michelle Pinelle,

for investing your time and energy into training me.

You didn't have to go the extra mile to mold a new graduate,

but you did. My nursing abilities are a reflection of

your teachings. I am forever grateful.

To Kerri Tillquist and Christina Lanzen,

for being the nurses who took care of my father

in his final hours.

The love, care, compassion, and knowledge you possessed

made me realize what kind of nurse I wanted to be.

Ever since, I've dedicated every day of my life

to being that person for someone else.

Quotes from the Minds and Hearts of Intensive Care Unit Nurses

"For many years I was strong technically, but it took becoming a patient myself to truly understand their vulnerability. I now know that everything matters: every big and every little thing!"

~ Meg Sakala

"Critical Care is one of those disciplines where exhilaration and terror live together simultaneously." ~Anonymous

"Never underestimate anything in the ICU. The moment you do is the moment you are losing the battle." ~Anonymous

"Critical Care humbles everyone. No matter how brilliant you are, the human body can always counter with something unforeseen."

~ Pamela Karakusis

"I love critical care nursing for the special impact we can have on a patient and/or their loved ones. In their greatest time of need they come to us, to lean into us for support and guidance, and all of our specialty nursing skills." ~Meg Sakala

"My favorite part of critical care is being able to ask my patient their name and hear them respond. We often don't get to hear our patient's voices." ~Pamela Karakusis

"I never thought I'd hold laughter and tears in the same regard, but now I do." ~Anonymous

"There's nothing harder than telling someone only time will tell. The fear and pain of not knowing is all-consuming." ~Anonymous

"Critical care makes you realize life and death waits for nothing."

~Anonymous

Table of Contents

Introduction

This project started in a completely organic fashion. I was experiencing nursing burnout and, to put it lightly, I was emotionally overwhelmed. Desperate to find a solution, I started exercising excessively. The exercise helped to a point but also resulted in utter exhaustion. The more tired I became, the more my turmoil got the better of me.

Being a part of the medical profession presents many challenges and honoring privacy practices is one that will always be relevant. Much of the work we do has to be left at the workplace. Our daily experiences are not appropriate dinner conversation, for many reasons, but primarily because it could violate patient privacy. You never know who you are eating dinner next to. It could be a family member of the person whose case you are discussing. Furthermore, medical events and stories are often shocking. Even if discussing my experiences with those outside the medical profession were permitted, it would be too heavy a burden for anyone not accustomed to the emotional toll and graphic nature of my job.

Given the fact that it isn't generally possible to try to ease my burnout by talking through my experiences with family or friends, I realized I needed to find another way to rid myself of this baggage I'd been carrying around. I needed an emotional detox. To accomplish this I started journaling. However, some of my sentiments were too difficult to put into words.

Having been an artistic person all my life, I began sketching what I could not express in writing. As the years progressed, something miraculous happened. I felt better! I was no longer burned out, but rather refreshed. Interestingly enough, during the same time period my cases had become increasingly complex, and I had taken on a leadership role with extra responsibilities and stress, but I was more able to deal with them. I noticed that I had become more deeply aware of myself and my feelings surrounding these subjects; but more importantly, I was now able to articulate and express them. With that in mind, I decided to assemble my thoughts into a collection of essays, letters, poems, and drawings dedicated to the realities nurses deal with every day. My hope was, and is, to honor the mental hardships and successes we experience within the nursing profession.

A Few Key Terms:

These two terms appear frequently throughout the book, so I've given clarifying information here for those who may not be familiar with medical terminology.

ICU: Intensive Care Unit; a unit in a hospital for dangerously ill or injured patients where they are constantly monitored.

Critical Care: A term to describe the type of care administered to patients who have dangerous and often life-threatening injury or illness. This is the type of care patients receive while in an intensive care unit.

Chapter 1: Critical Care

Critical care reminds me of the ocean. It's always flowing and constantly changing; a force that's unpredictable and vast. There is peace and beauty intermixed with distress and uncertainty. The nurses within this setting are, without a doubt, the bridge between medicine and humanity. In critical care our connections become increasingly important since there is often a "man vs machine" dynamic. We have all the benefits of modern technology and healthcare advancements at our fingertips. Such resources allow us to save many lives, but they can also make the environment frightening and uncomfortable. While medical professionals are well acclimated to this environment, it can be all too easy to forget that patients and families often feel as if they have stepped onto another planet. Simultaneously, they are experiencing high levels of physical and emotional stress, which only adds insult to injury.

We as ICU nurses live within this environment every day. It's what we do. Our world revolves around being comfortable in uncomfortable situations. The question is, how does one find peace and comfort in the midst of chaos? In theory this may seem simple, but it is actually one of the most intricate parts of what we do because every patient, family, and situation is unique. Our interactions, regardless of how big or small, have to be genuine. They have to come from a place deep inside ourselves, so that we can identify and relate with the myriad emotions and experiences of others. We have all been sick, scared, loved, and felt lost. We have all been confused, tired, angry, and overwhelmed. It's part of life and what makes us human. There are moments in everyone's life when we simply need someone to be there; in nursing we get to be the ones lending our strength. It's truly a powerful process. We cannot save every person, but we can be present for each and every moment.

We were all motivated and inspired to go into this profession for a reason. When we connect with who we are and why we love what we do, that awareness projects itself into our interactions. Our passion and love for nursing as well as for our patients transcends through any situation or setting. It's an aura that patients and families can feel, leading to the creation of trust, which then leads to confidence in care. The relationship fostered by that process is impactful because it's real and it is imperative for quality medical care. Life is all about passion and loving something or someone; nursing elevates that by loving all people.

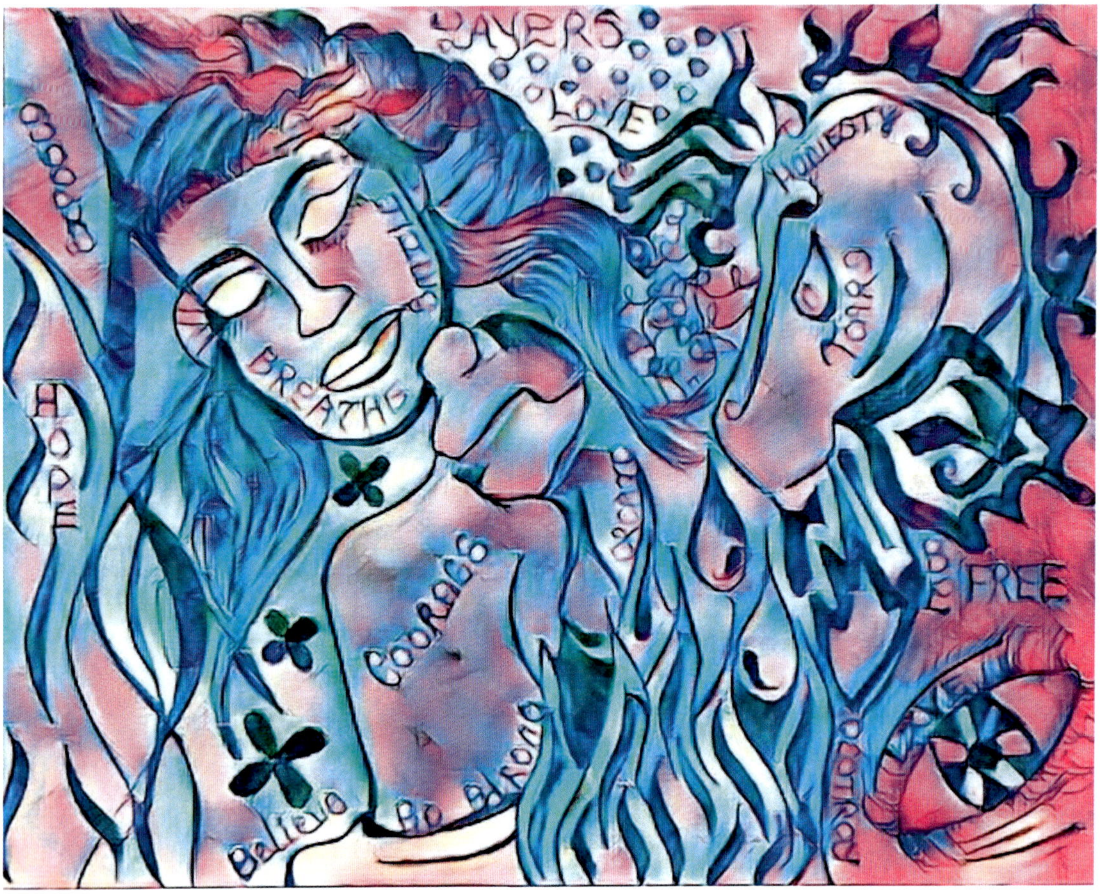
LOVE
HONESTY
BREATHE
HOPE
BE FREE

Empathy

One of the key qualities for every nurse to possess is empathy. Demonstrating empathy may seem simplistic and is frequently written off as insignificant, but nothing could be further from the truth. We nurses are confronted with situations every day that make us question our own humanity and ethics while requiring us to open our minds to the perspectives of others. All the while, we may disagree with someone's life choices or even be struggling with the moral principles at play. It's a fine balance because having empathy doesn't mean we disrespect ourselves or the decisions of others, but rather that we practice love and understanding within a dynamic and diverse set of issues. The mental and emotional toll can become all too real, affecting longevity in this profession.

As I mentioned earlier, writing and artistic expression have been my outlets. I often write through the eyes of my patients to express what they cannot. Some people have viewed my pieces as innovative and beautiful; others have described them as dark, disturbing, and even morbid. Moving forward, regardless of where your heart lands on this spectrum, I'm glad if my work makes you feel something, because that's really what empathy is all about.

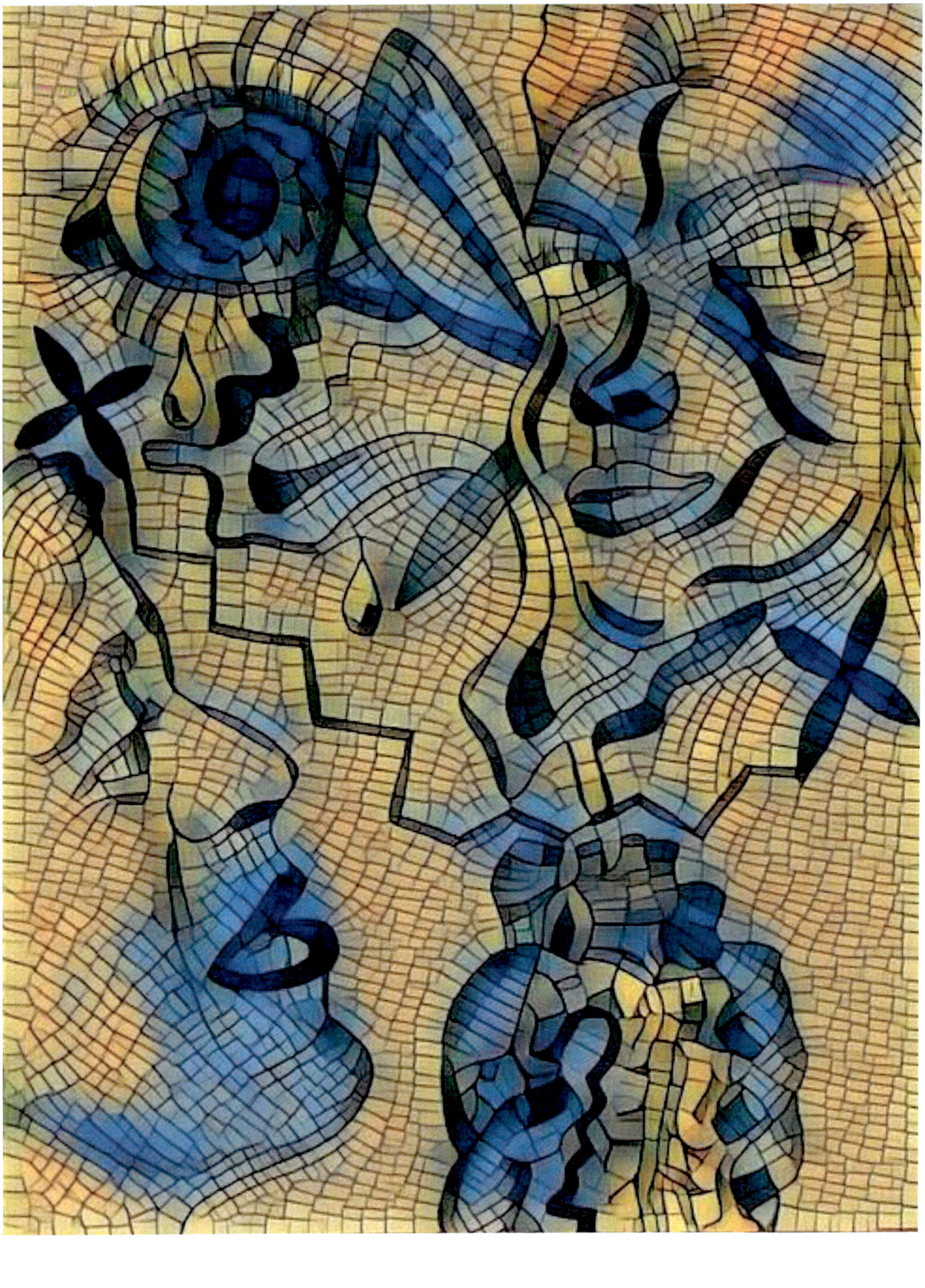

Integrity

Talk to me about love, talk to me about money, talk to me about sex, talk to me about anything as long as what you have to say is truthful and real. I may disagree with your ideas or opinions, but I'll never fault you for honesty. When did we all become so afraid to talk to one another? Working in the ICU, there's simply no time for inauthenticity. The experience is raw, needs are immediate, and interactions are often emotionally intimate. I have the utmost respect for the honesty of this atmosphere. With such high stakes for the patients and the intensity of the situation for their loved ones, integrity is vital. No one–and I mean no one–is going to trust their life to you without it.

Cardiac ICU

There's an unmistakable force looming as you wait for your open-heart surgery patient. The anticipation alone leaves you breathless, but there is a presence in the air that you cannot place or name. You wonder if it's your own thoughts, the desire to help fix what is broken, to restore a life that could be lost. Maybe it's your devotion to giving someone back to their family. The truth is you have no idea how this day is going to end. The volatility is somewhat exciting, but it also makes you hesitate.

There will be opportunity to use the skills you've spent hours perfecting. The chance to tap into the mind you've endlessly trained is a source of thrill. However, the devil lurking in the dark is fear. The cold, hard reality is this: if complications are too great, you might not be able to save the patient. You know that when their heart bleeds, yours will too. This moment, before you begin, will be your last quiet one before the storm. You will have to trust yourself and take solace in the fact that regardless of the outcome, you will be present. As you see the team roll down the hallway with your patient, you take a deep breath. It's time for you to do what you were born to do, because one thing is certain; you were meant to deal with matters of the heart.

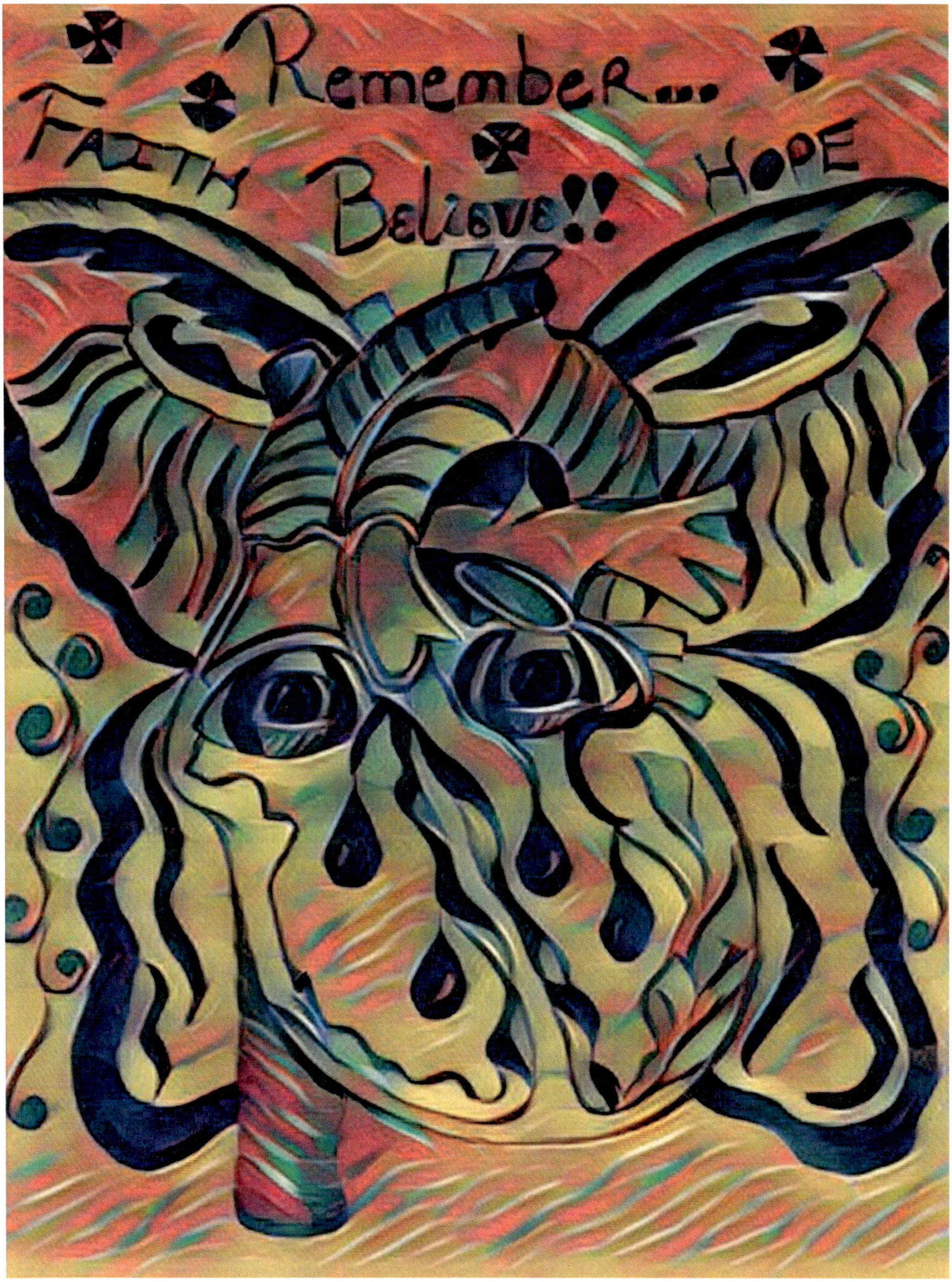
Remember...
FAITH
HOPE
Believe!!

Get It Together

If you are going to work in the ICU, you have to be able to handle the pressure. It's a job that requires you to be "on" all the time and to utilize all of your brain power. You're fighting a battle, so to speak, with the human body; trying to get it to work with you rather than against you. It's essential to be three moves ahead and to manage the attack to the best of your ability. All those memes referring to critical care nurses as "rigidly organized control freaks" are completely accurate. Sorry everyone! The truth hurts sometimes. We are trained to be exacting in our observations, to think of everything, because if we don't, people die.

The next essay, Intensity (p. 13), focuses on pressure. We all handle intense situations differently. I've found that critical care nurses have an interesting relationship with stress. We thrive under pressure and often seek out situations and assignments that test our ability to manage not only complex processes, but also our own emotions. The goal of an ICU nurse is to be the calmest person in the room. You need to possess a sense of urgency, yet be in control of your emotions because once you lose control of yourself, you lose control of the situation.

Intensity

I love the heat. There's nothing quite like it. It's an intensity that plays by its own rules. As the temperature rises, possessive, it approaches slowly so that, at first, it evades notice. But soon, it burns to make its presence known. Navigating its paradoxical nature is compelling; warmth is pleasant, but too much heat will become restrictive. So you settle, feeling the temperature rise, embracing the expected constriction and welcoming the emotions that are revealed. Fully aware, you stare down the animal as it approaches, unsure of your fate. It's unclear whether this standoff is purging toxins or innocence. You are bleeding from every pore. The air is thick and vice-like. You watch your chest move violently in and out. Each breath labored. Merciless and covetous are the forces that come for you. Trembling, the corners of your mouth turn up. Only one question remains: Who can handle the heat?

Chapter 2: Trauma In The ICU

I must warn you: throughout this book there are many passages that are heavy on trauma because I reside with it daily. However, it's important to note that tragedy happens to us all. It's an experience to which just about everyone can relate. So while some of the content may be distressing, please proceed, because there is great value in allowing ourselves to acknowledge whatever may be stirred within us by confronting trauma. Being surrounded by heartbreak and devastation always takes a toll. The day it doesn't, the day you lose compassion, is the day you know you are done.

Critical care is riddled with cases that touch our hearts and even leave us with emotional scars, but I wouldn't have it any other way. I've become a better person as a result of this work and I've gained a deeper appreciation for life than I ever thought possible. Ultimately, critical care chose me, not the other way around; I will always be grateful for it. You are about to encounter a special case which embodies everything intensive care unit nursing is about. It will stay with me forever.

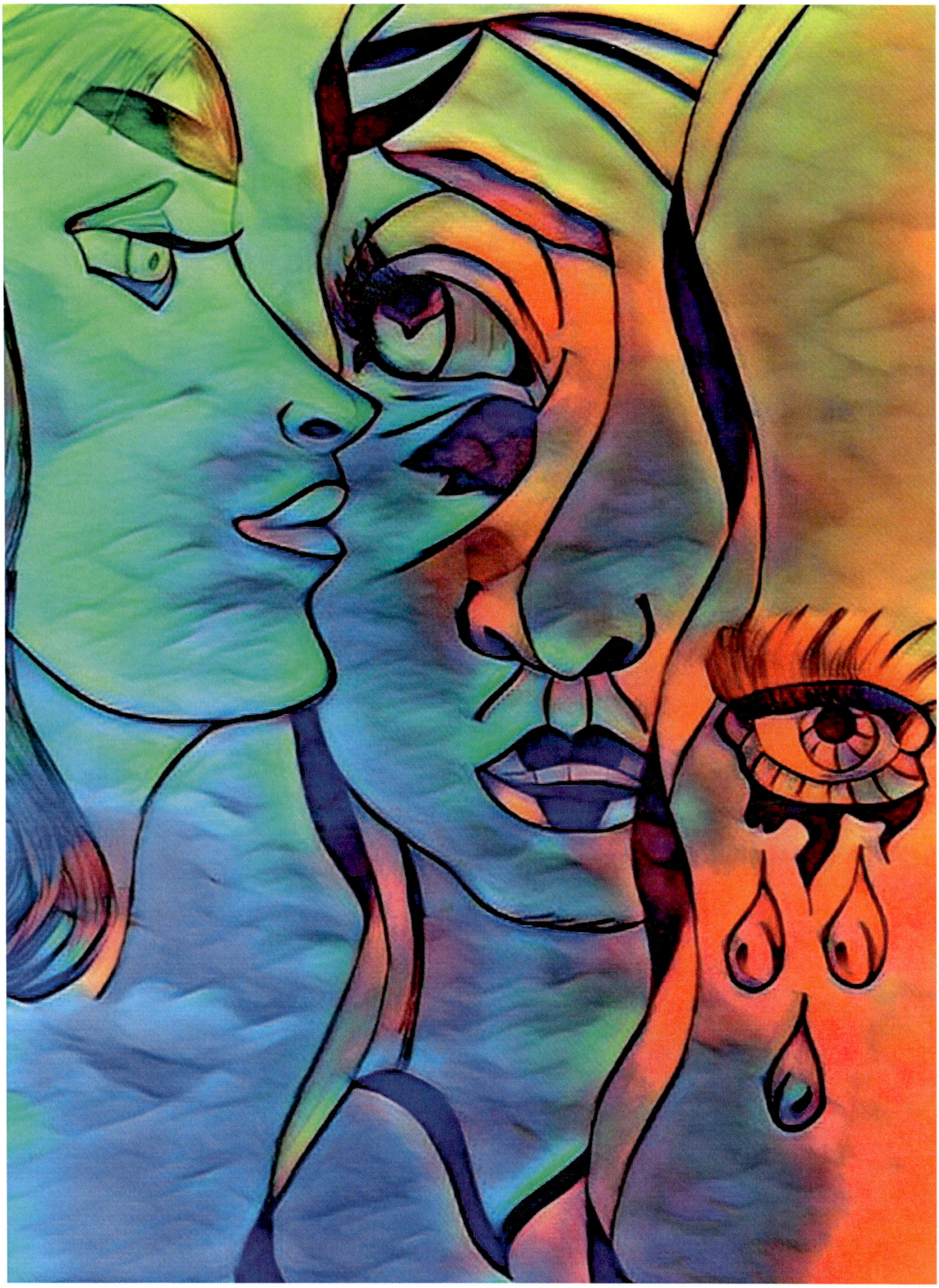

Burnt Depression/Stand By Me

You often hear stories about those patients that left a lasting impression on the nurses and physicians who cared for them. You listen to the profound impact those patients have had on the careers and even the lives of those professionals. Truth be told, I had never had a case that I couldn't let go of, until this one.

This patient was a handsome and vibrant young man who had decided to light himself on fire! His exact reasons for doing so will never be known, but a detailed history of depression and a strained relationship with his family were possible catalysts for his terrible choice. Burned extensively everywhere except for his feet, he came to me as my patient on ECMO (extracorporeal membrane oxygenation/extracorporeal life support). This is a machine that transports your blood out of the body and acts as an artificial lung and/or heart. It's the most extreme measure we can implement to attempt to save a life and this young man was, without a doubt, fighting for his. I vividly remember getting wind of his story and instantly being flooded with emotions. I knew immediately that I had to take care of him.

With another ECMO already running that day, I was the only available ECMO-certified nurse on-site. He would have been mine by default, but had that not been the case, I still would have fought to take care of him. As a mother of four, I couldn't help but think about how I'd feel if this were my son, my baby. Complicating my thoughts was the fact that my own teenage son was also dealing with depression and there were many days when I worried about what I might find upon returning home. I even called my son before receiving this patient to tell him how much I loved him. After our conversation, it was time to put those feelings aside because I knew my focus had to be all on this young man. It was time to do what I do best. As he arrived to me it was clear this battle was going to be uphill. I needed to give him every ounce of my energy and even so, it might not be enough.

Regardless of whatever unknowns the day might hold, I immediately made a promise to this young man. I told him I wouldn't leave his side, and in that moment, my co-workers were making the same promise to stand by *my* side. People frequently ask me how I do what I do, and my answer is beautifully simple. I am able to do this job because of my co-workers, people I also count as friends. I am able to do this job because I have an amazing group of individuals on my team who support me. When faced with cases like this one, we rarely think of ourselves. It becomes vital that we are all taking care of each other so that we can form the unbreakable support network that will envelop our patient. Taking care of this young man really made a lasting impression on me, driving home the point that we need that vital support network in order to administer the care and attention that our patients deserve.

This particular day I stood in a stiflingly hot room, gowned, gloved, and masked, while exerting all of my physical and emotional energy for twelve hours trying to save this young man. My friends hydrated me, fed me, hugged me, and offered any kind of support I needed. There aren't many professions with this kind of camaraderie and it's exactly what got me through the day. It's what we do as nurses–we save people. Sometimes we save each other too.

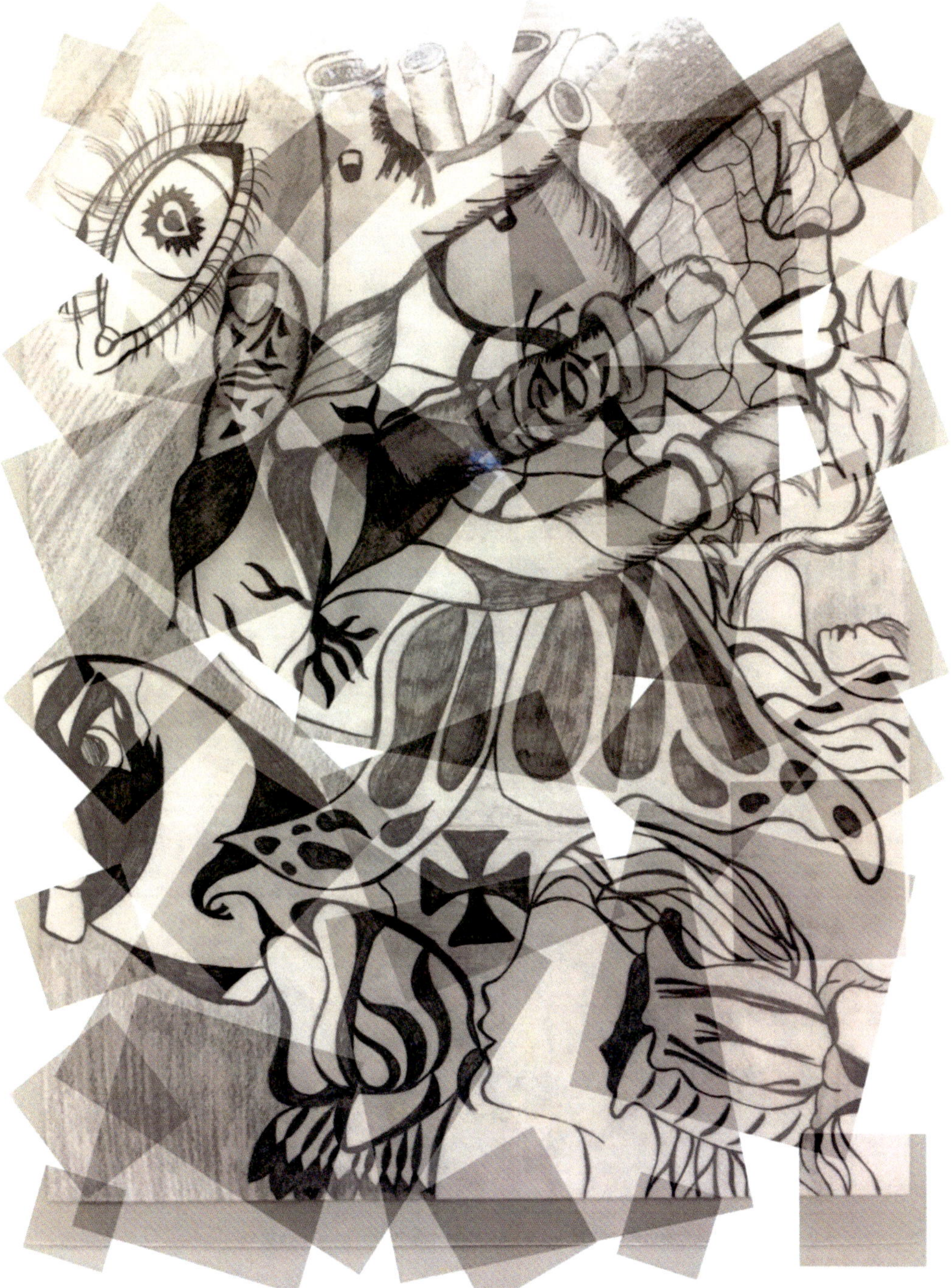

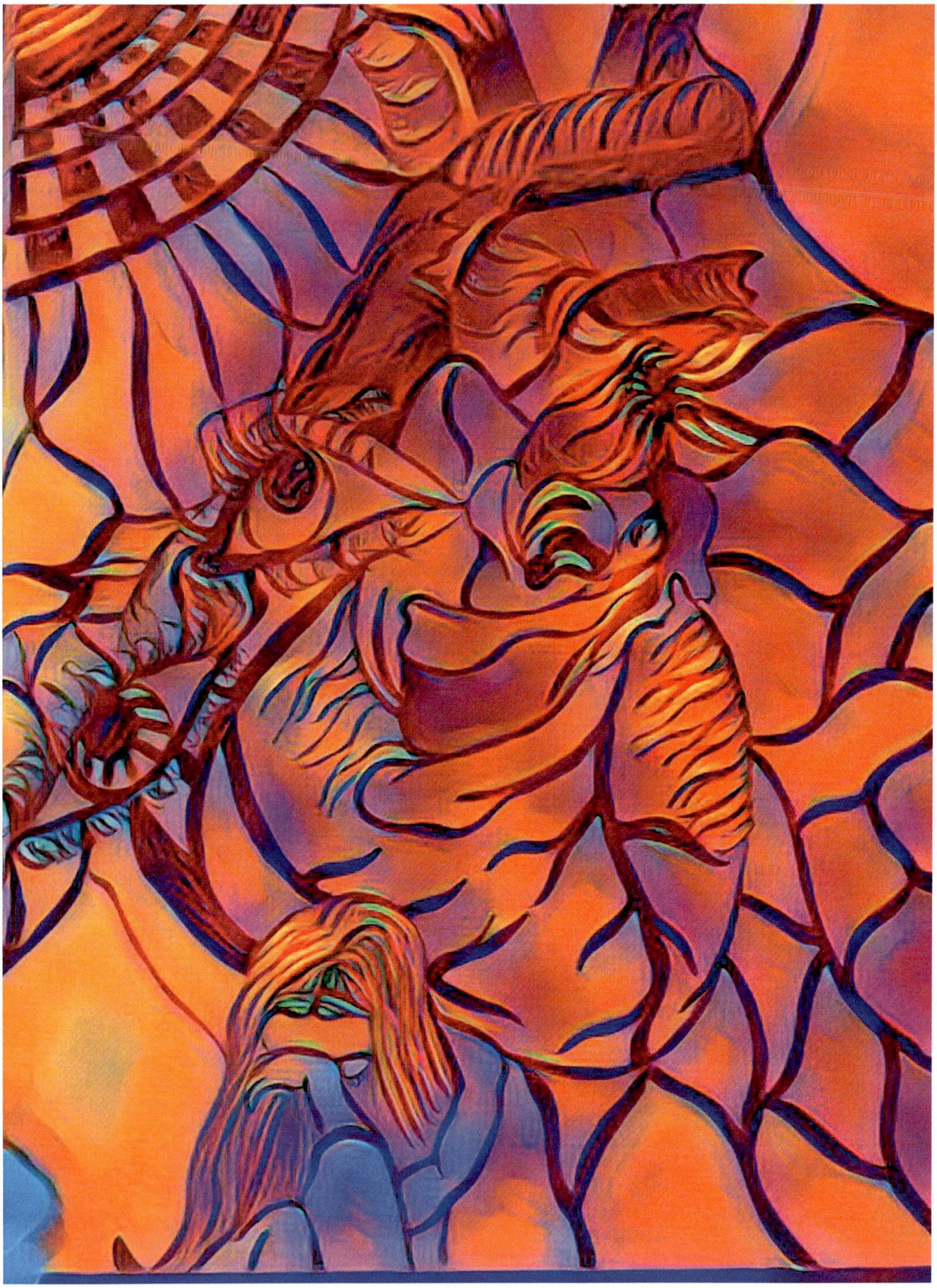

The Yin And Yang: Duality Of Good And Evil

Trauma is awkwardly revealing. It will unveil all of the forces at work; those functioning harmoniously and also those in direct opposition to one another. Therefore, I wanted to make sure this next painting (p. 22) depicted struggle and sadness, but also hope, because all three often exist in the same space. Experiences shape who we are and our lives are a fragile balance between that which helps us grow and that which holds us back. So, at first glance do you see the good, the evil, or both?

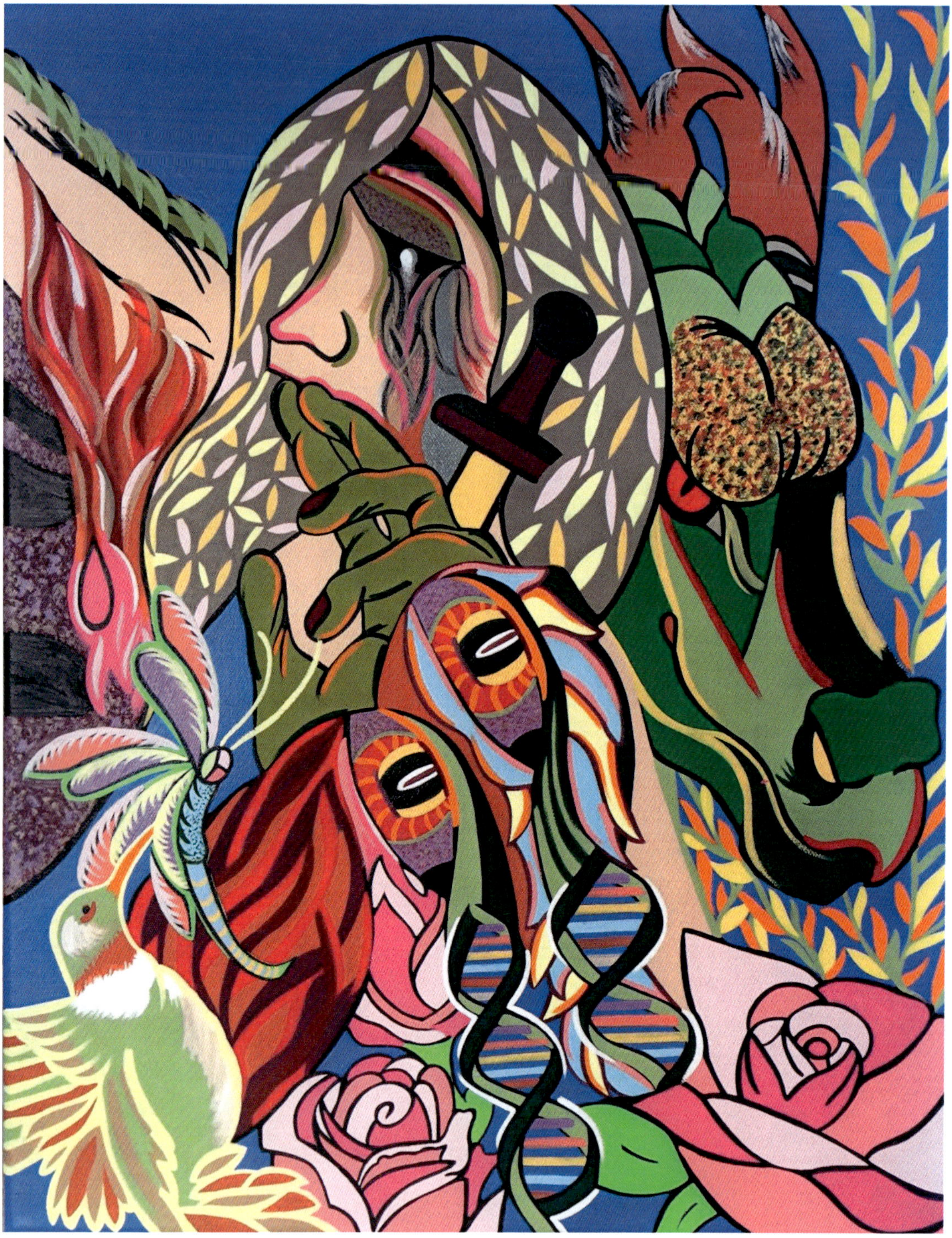

Transformation: The Way Forward

We are all mosaics in the sense that our identities are made up of thousands of pieces; experiences, perceptions, emotions, and so much more. Now, how that all fits together is up to each individual. And sometimes, the way it all fits together must change. Throughout my career, I have watched so many patients and families adapting to what I refer to as “a new normal”. I think the hardest part of the process for most is realizing that transformation takes time. Recovering from critical illness or injury is a lengthy process and it can start to feel like nothing is ever going to improve. At the beginning, people don’t yet realize that although life from this point on may be different, it can be just as rich as before. When I talk to patients and their families about these transformations, I often use an example such as caterpillars turning into butterflies or waiting for the seasons to change every year. Both phenomena take time, but they are well worth the wait.

The transformations I’ve seen so many going through reminds me of how we experience art. Truly appreciating a piece of art means understanding that the experience is not static. Beauty lies within dimension and color is a dynamic visual perception. One’s impression of a piece of art can change due to a number of factors, including when and under what conditions the art piece is seen. My hope is that people are able to see themselves as a work of art too;

one that is still being refined. There is nothing more important than people understanding that their mosaic can change and yet still be beautiful. Throughout the healing process and through all of their transformations, people need to know that they are still loved and valued within this dynamic, dimensional, beautiful life.

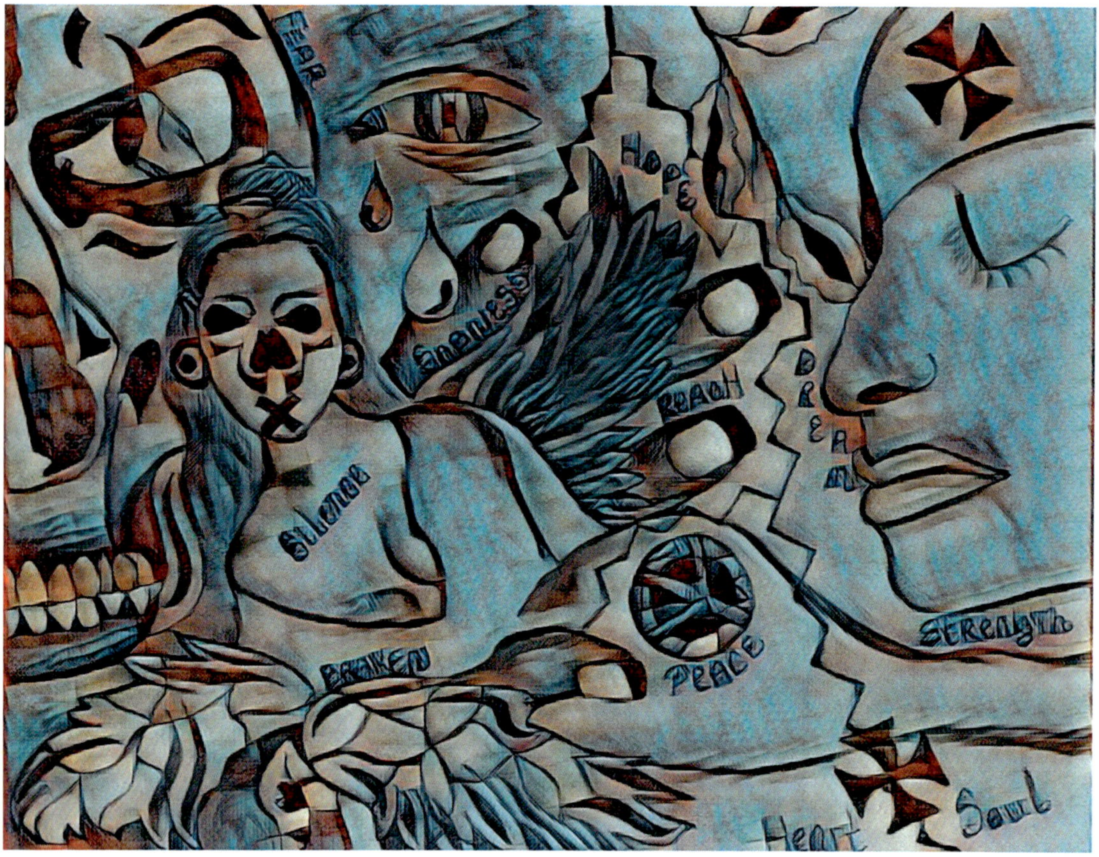

Chapter 3: Loss And Grief

Loss is complicated. At one point in my life I thought time would heal all wounds, but truthfully, I lacked an understanding of grief because I personally had not experienced it yet. Within the intensive care unit, loss is a part of our world. We are forced to acknowledge and embrace the unspoken reality; death is a component of life. With that, I must say I'm thankful to have been a support for so many people during their own loss, because I'll never forget the nurses who were there for mine.

Years ago, I chose to take my father off of life support after he suffered a massive brain hemorrhage due to a glioblastoma stage 4 (a deadly kind of brain tumor). The diagnosis itself was a shock and I still hadn't processed the finality that came with his disease before having to make that irreversible decision. I remember shrieking wildly and bawling uncontrollably. The disbelief overtook me. What had I done? He was gone. All I could think in that moment was, "I killed him". I frantically paced and chanted this statement over and over until finally collapsing onto the floor. What happened next was my saving grace.

One of his nurses came over and sat with me. She held onto me as if to shelter me from my own thoughts. In that moment I hated myself for deciding his fate. Every ounce of me believed my big, strong father was going to suddenly wake up and prove science wrong, but he didn't. My whole body was numb, shaking, and the entire time his nurse never let me go. For some time as I sat there, everything was a complete blur. What I do remember is finally being overcome by a sense of peace. When my awareness of my surroundings came flooding back, that nurse was still there. Without saying a single word, she got me through those moments of absolute despair and never left my side. Her compassion is permanently etched on my heart.

To this day, that memory is a reminder of why I love nursing. Granted, I've loved medicine since I was a little girl, but the day I lost my father is the day I really fell in love with the people who choose the profession. Looking back over all the years my father has been gone, I still miss him just as much. Sometimes it hurts like it did the day he died. The difference now is that I'm not ashamed to admit it. Loss is complicated and difficult to endure, but there is beauty in all of our emotions, including grief.

These next few pieces are ones that I've written over the years to celebrate my father. They've helped me process my own grief and are a reflection of the healing process that so many of us must face. So, read on, in honor of those we've loved and lost, the ones we couldn't save, and those to whom we've brought some measure of peace.

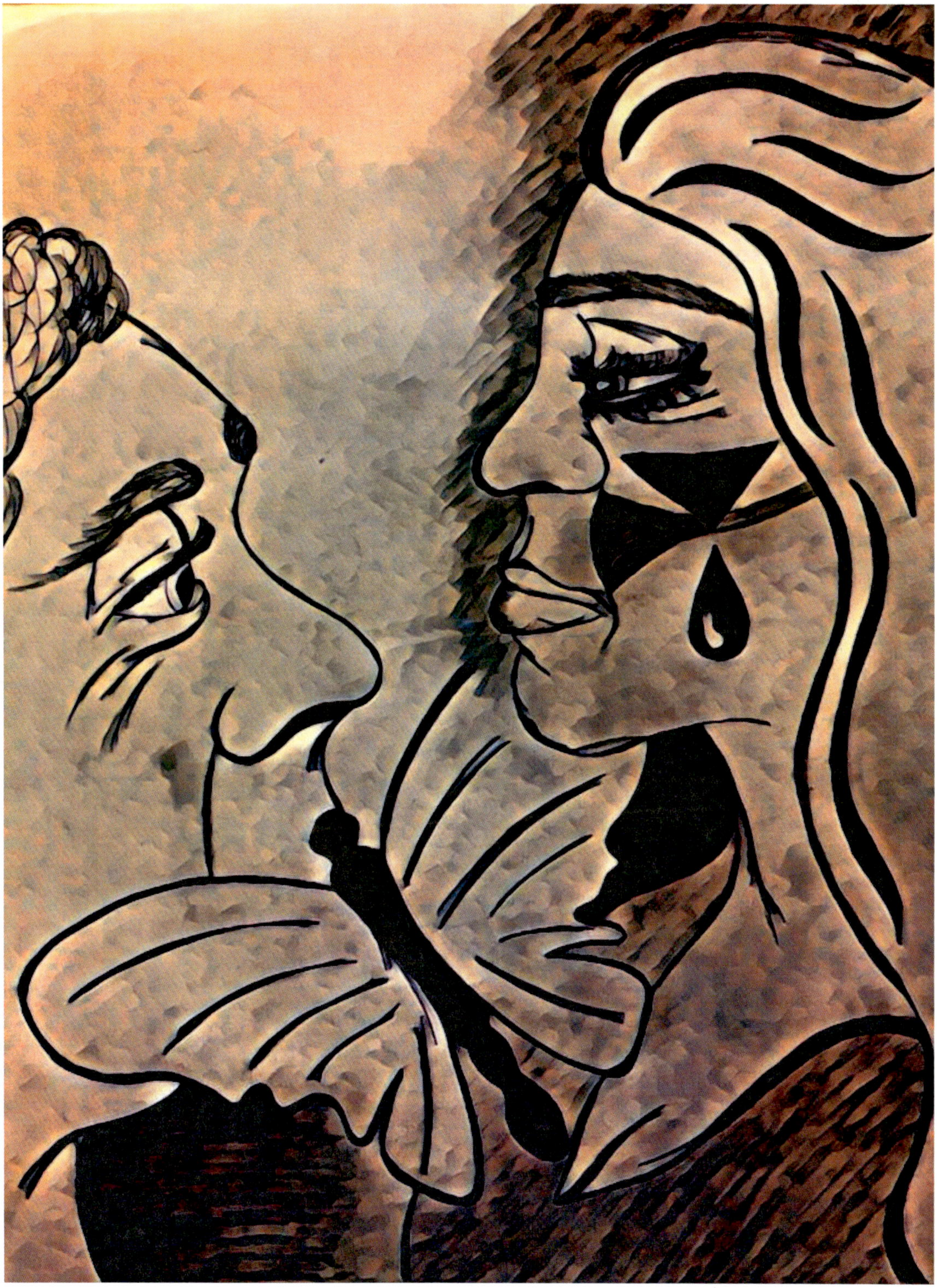

A Daughter's Remembrance

Dad,

It's hard to believe you've been gone for so long. Seven years to be exact and I still miss you every day. There are so many things I'd like to tell you, so many things I'd like to say. I've always been a Daddy's girl at heart and not much has changed. I love that you used to buy me roses for no reason, always red. Some of my other favorite memories are our late-night chess matches and your love of the written word. The dictionary was your all-time favorite book; that still makes me laugh! We used to drive for hours to little "hole-in-the-wall" restaurants with the intention of finding a "diamond in the rough". The chance of food poisoning was fifty-fifty, but it was part of the adventure, so we didn't care. And of course, there was the infamous Christmas tree you left up all year long, partly to irritate Yiayia (my Greek grandmother), but mostly because you loved the magic of the holiday season.

You know you changed my life forever when you held my hand as we walked over the bridge that connected the parking garage to the hospital where you worked as an infectious disease doctor. I didn't want you to go to work that day. At only five years old, I wanted you to play princess with me instead. You said, "Honey, people can't help when they get sick. They get sick on their birthdays and on holidays. I need to try to make them better so they can go home."

Ever since that day I've wanted to be just like you. So, walk these long, white halls with me again today, but this time Dad, I'll bring you the roses! Love you, forever and always!

-Pamela

Dedicated to: Peter H. Karakusis, MD

March 29, 1951–November 8, 2010

"Life is all about the experience, so be safe and I love you!"— Dr. Karakusis

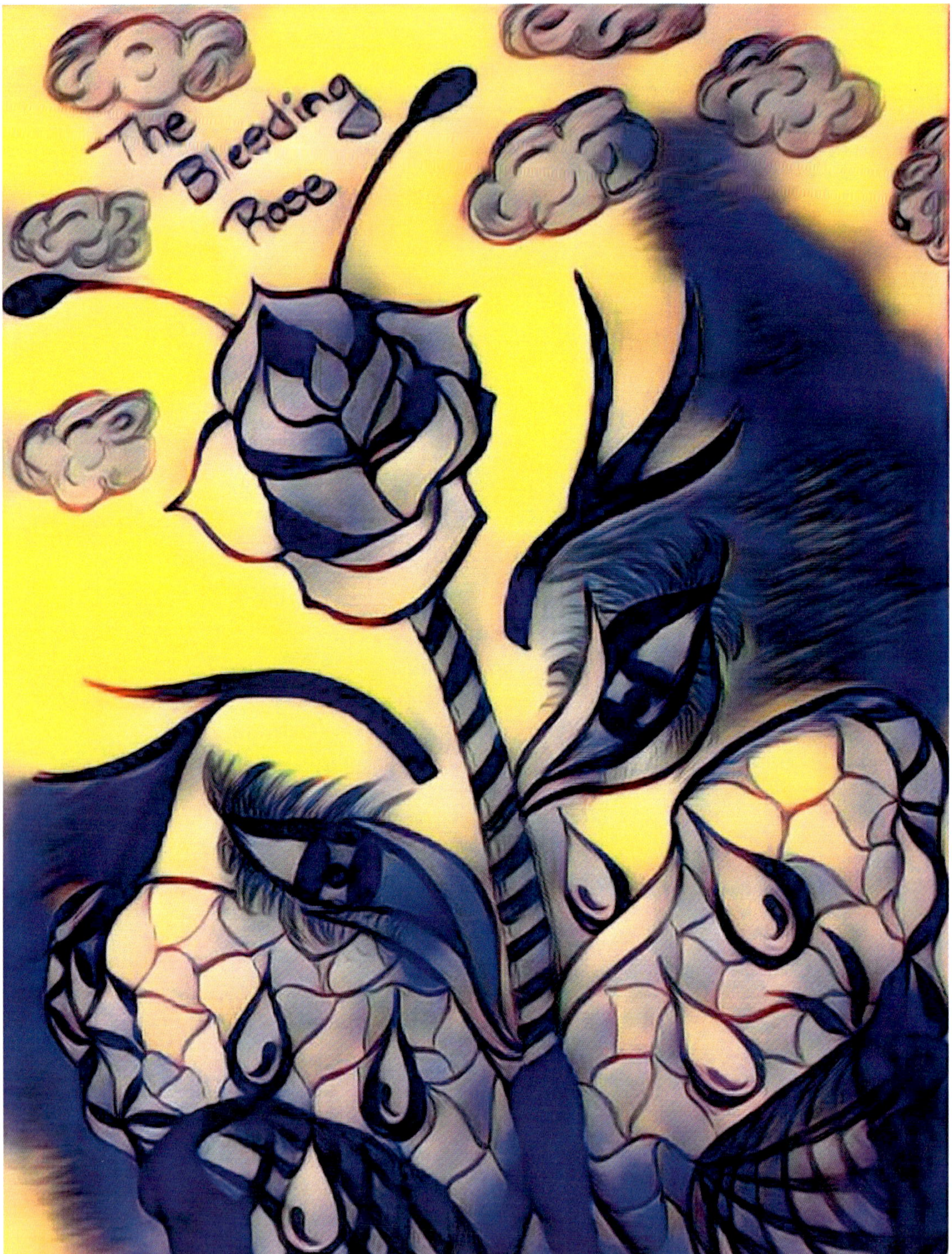
The Bleeding Rose

Wishing Upon A Star

As my father's illness progressed, there were many days when his conversations were plagued by confusion. Regardless of his mental state, I loved and treasured every minute I had with him. On one of his good days he looked up at me and told me that I looked sad. I was sitting in a chair next to his bed, blankly staring out the window. There was nothing outside except the street I grew up on, but I was envisioning him mowing the lawn or shoveling the snow. He was always such a character and chores took him hours because he just had to make the biggest snow pile or mow designs into the grass. Along with all of those wonderful memories came the realization that my father would not have another summer and might not even see the next forecasted snow; he'd caught me in this moment without my brave face. He asked me to come sit next him on the bed, which I gladly did. Then he asked me if I was going to be okay. At the time I did not know what to say. I had no idea if I was going to be alright or if I was strong enough to watch him deteriorate. Instinctively, wanting to avoid distressing him, I told him not to worry about me. He was the one who was dying and should not be focusing on me; I should be focusing on him.

My father then spoke words to me that I will always hold dear. He even wrote them down for me to remember after he passed. I've spent many hours literally holding these words in my hands:

I'll miss your face and beautiful mind. When you're lonely, meet me under the stars because that's where you'll find me waiting for you with open arms, and never forget I'll always be with you. So please don't be sad. I want you to laugh and dance in the rain and go after your dreams, because I promise you, I'll still be there!

Love, Dad ❤

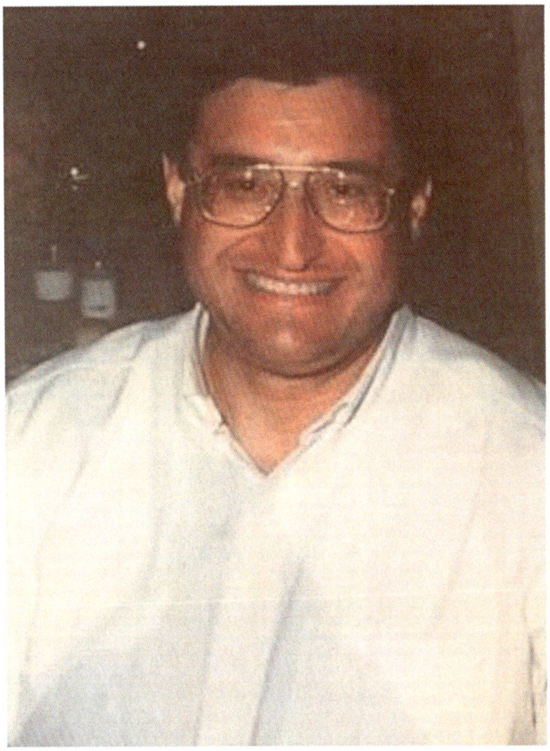

Peter Karakusis, M.D.

*Note: One of his favorite things to do, outside of work, was try new restaurants.
Here he is in the late 1990s doing just that.
His smile could light up an entire room.*

My Father's Heart

Dad,

As I write this, it's been eight years since we last spoke while you held my hand. I'll never forget you sleeping on my bedroom floor when I was sick or checking for monsters in the house to ease my fears. I must admit, this happened well into my twenties, but you never cared. You always came when I needed you. Those memorable late-night powwows, coke floats, and your must-have vanilla bean Frappuccino with a shot of chocolate; all hold a special place in my heart. That being said, our last conversation could be my favorite memory, because it showed your big, teddy-bear-heart; but that conversation will always be just for us!

-Pamela

My Light In The Sky

Dad,

It's been nine years since that awful day; one that I'll never forget. I had to let you go. It was the hardest thing I've ever done. I couldn't imagine my life without you. What was this girl going to do without her dad? To this day, I like to imagine that you are amongst the stars. Every night, I find the brightest one in the sky and tell you how much I love you. Sometimes I wonder if I told you that enough while you were here. I always thought we had more time. I always thought there'd be another conversation. But truth be told, regardless of whether I can see your smile or hear your voice, I know you are with me. Thank you for being my bright and beautiful star shining down on me always! I love you Dad, forever and always.

-Pamela

Our Angels

Unfortunately, we see a lot of youth vanish before their time. I can't even imagine what it's like to lose a child. In a perfect world parents wouldn't bury their kids. In the medical profession, we see everything from accidents to unfortunate life choices to singular mistakes that end up costing the ultimate price. The reality is that you can only teach your kids so much and at some point, their decisions become their own. As parents we're left hoping they make good ones. Regardless of age, our kids will always be our babies. They are treasured souls, but ones we cannot always keep close. They are meant to grow up and fly away from us, just not as angels.

The poem that follows was inspired by a young patient and his mother. We had all been casual acquaintances prior to his becoming my patient, but were brought closer together during one of life's very difficult moments. After the young man passed away, his mother told me she was going to visit the cemetery all the time to be close to him. She and I ended up having many conversations that impacted me greatly.

Out of respect for their privacy, I will not disclose any details, but I will say that our conversations were the caveat for this next piece. I was intentional about simplicity and subtlety in the composition, because writing about someone visiting their child's grave demands careful handling.

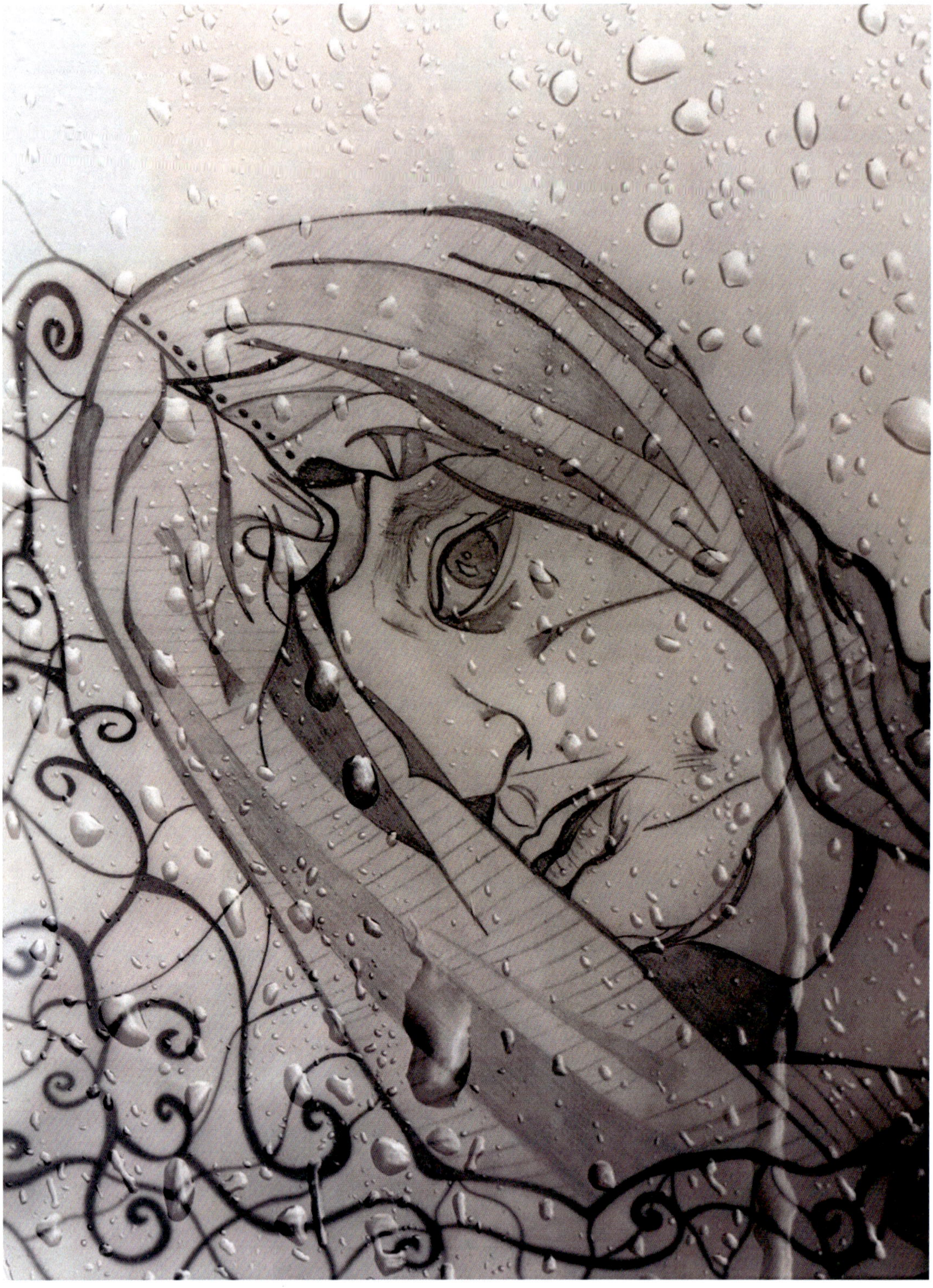

The Grave Sight

Mother can you see me?

I am not a boy anymore, for I am a man.

I know I have been far away from home, but I have returned.

Please don't cry.

Let me wipe away your tears.

I am here with you just as you are here with me.

Look up and see your son.

My hand is resting on your face.

Can you feel me?

Listen closely and let my voice guide you.

Remember the ocean and why I love it so.

You can hear its heart and feel its soul from miles away.

Can you hear me?

Shells are pieces of the ocean's heart,

scattered along the shore they rest, sometimes hidden, but they are not gone.

So look for me!

I am holding you in my arms.

Try to breathe even though it hurts.

Put your hand to your heart.

I am here!

Tears are wearing lines on your cheeks.

I will kiss your forehead, as you have always kissed mine.

I'm your angel to guide you.

Can you sense my presence?

Don't doubt your instincts.

Have faith and believe in me.

Yes, mother it's your son.

I love you with all that I am.

We will be together again someday,

but for now, reach out with your hand.

You can touch my name and touch me!

Chapter 4: Therapeutic Meditation And The Darkest Hours

Meditation has become a huge part of my life. It helps me relax and regroup, especially after some long and emotionally draining shifts. To be honest, I wasn't always a fan of meditation. I didn't think it could help me with what I was going through. I'd tried to create a box for myself, to contain my mental and emotional exhaustion. Eventually I realized that I had only succeeded in shutting the door on solutions. I'd closed myself off, but why? To this day I believe it was because I had some extremely raw emotions to process and a part of me was afraid to confront those emotions. No one wants to rub salt in wounds. However, ignoring everything wasn't helping either. Therefore, I decided it was time to invest more in myself and my well-being. It was time to dare to be different. I was pleasantly surprised by the process of coming to greater self-awareness. Your mind can take you wherever you want to go and when mind, body, and spirit connect as one, enlightenment follows.

The next few entries highlight some of my experiences of nursing shifts that seemed to come from hell. They are the darkest hours, both figuratively and (sometimes) literally. Every medical professional knows what I'm talking about. You just have to hang on for dear life. Those are the days when all you can manage is to hydrate and even dinner will probably be liquid because you don't have time to chew! And yes, I'd like to confirm the rumor as true, nurses sometimes go without using the bathroom for twelve hours because there just isn't time. Food for thought!

Hell Hath No Fury Like The Night Shift

Note: At the facility where I work, the majority of patient admissions happen during the night shift. This means that there can be an overwhelming number of critically ill patients and not always enough beds to accommodate them. As the Clinical Nurse Coordinator, I am forced to play chess with people. I must make quick decisions about which patients are well enough to be moved out of the ICU in order to make room for those patients who must remain in critical care. It can really begin to seem like the nighttime contains some dark magical power that promotes illness and injury, and drives the poor souls in its clutches to my doorstep.

The night is menacing and lawless. You watch and actively participate in the pandemonium, trying to restore order. The time has come for evil, mystery, and fear to run wild within the human body. The phrase "naked and afraid" comes to mind, but it takes on a whole new meaning. When a stretcher lands in the unit, your patient is often both of those things, perhaps literally but very often subconsciously. The hours pass and the patients keep piling in, each one sicker than the last.

The battle persists until the much-welcomed sunrise. Part of you doesn't want to leave because you are invested in lives that may hang in the balance at that very moment, but the other part of you desperately needs a reprieve. So, you walk the knife-edge, forging ahead in spite of misgivings. The journey to your car seems endless. An internal battle is ensuing. The uncertainty of what you might find upon returning for your next shift overtakes your thoughts. The guardian existing within you cannot let go, but you leave anyway. There are multiple loves in your life, and now is the time to return to those outside of medicine.

The fresh smell of the early morning air is the only part of the drive home you remember. Slowly, in a slightly uncoordinated fashion, you steer yourself toward the shower. Most mornings you grant your mind permission to rest. However, today might be different. The warmth within the shower walls creates comfort and as you relax, you feel yourself crying. Maybe it's because you're tired, maybe it's because you're overwhelmed, or maybe it's because life and death were in your hands last night. There was no time to process or rationalize amidst the utter chaos.

There was the mother for whom you performed CPR (cardiopulmonary resuscitation), the teenager who shattered his body and possibly his life, the man without a face, and so many others who entered the battle with you. You wouldn't want it any other way because helping others is your life. This moment alone is simply your much-needed emotional release. You fight for the well-being of others yet sometimes forget about your own. The tears remind you that it's okay to be vulnerable and they bring you a sense of inner peace. This is your opportunity to let go. You cannot carry everyone's pain. As the weight lifts, you remember how proud you are of yourself and what you do. You love it and a smile comes to your face. You get to do it all again tomorrow and that's a beautiful thing, but for now you must sleep.

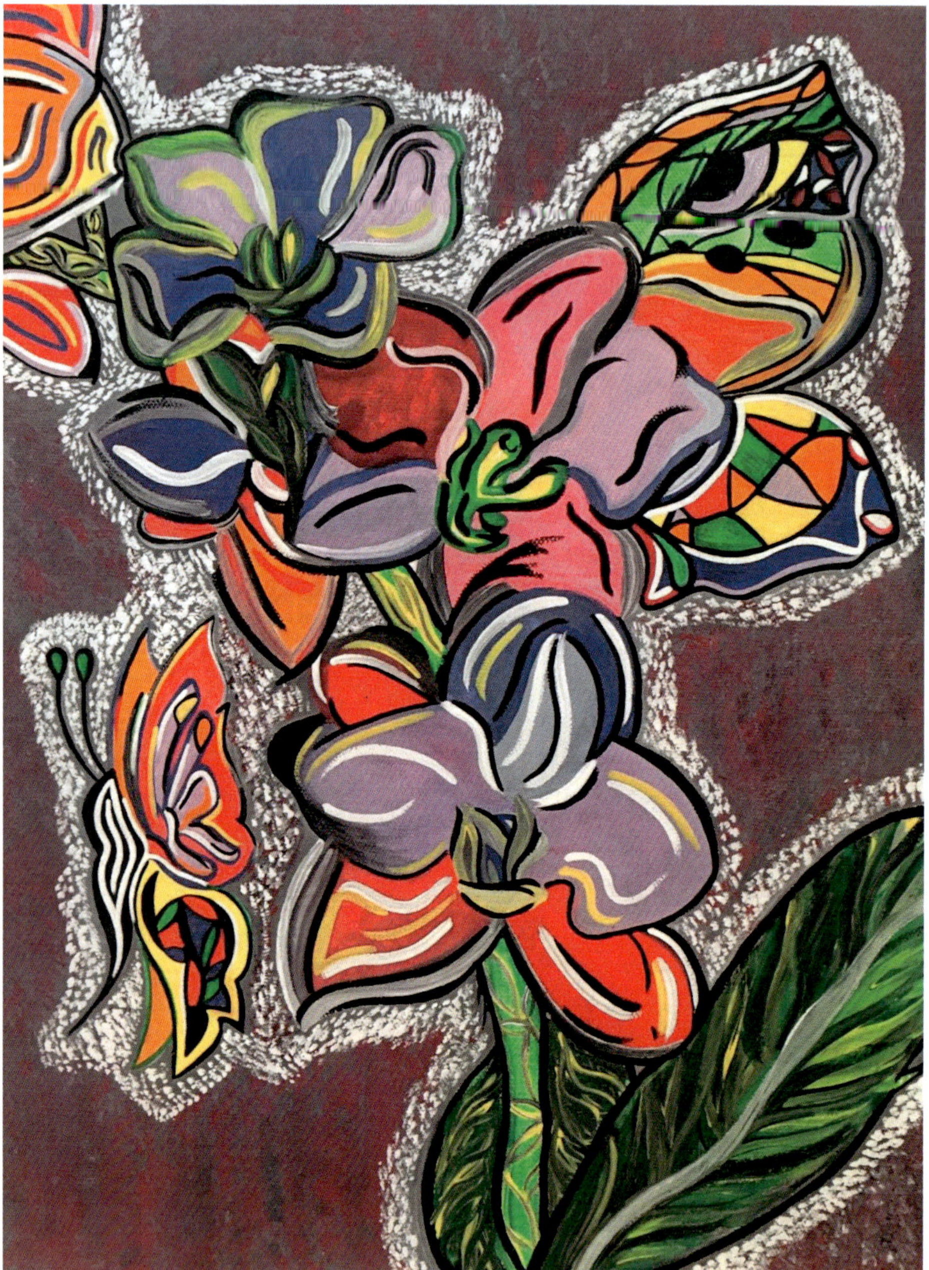

Let Me Introduce You...

I am about to introduce you to the "gentleman's monster"; a creative term for a vampire. This creature is known for being charming and debonair on the surface, yet ruthless in his true purpose. A night shift at the hospital is often referred to as the "vampire shift" for its striking similarity to this mythical being. The unpredictability of vampires after dark parallels the environment of the hospital at night. Working night shift for many years, I have had an up-close-and-personal interaction with how the world changes after dark. It is not uncommon to feel extra pressure during these solitary shifts. You are your patient's lifeline while the rest of the world sleeps. The essay that follows, entitled The Gentleman's Monster (p. 48), captures the psychological effects of the night shift. Like a vampire, you are awake during the lonely night hours and sleeping during the day. While the rest of the world sleeps, you must be on top of your game, administering care for a wide range of complex cases with less overall support from a reduced nighttime staff. The stress can make you question your career choice and even, at times, your own sanity.

The Gentleman's Monster

Sometimes I wonder why I do this job. It welcomes pain, sadness, and tears into my world. You're left all alone in the dark to manage a storm while the rest of the world retains an innocence you wish you could get back. But then again, you don't want it, because your perspective is like a black pearl; rare and unique and definitely not for everyone. You realize what you wish for instead is understanding from others, because you feel forgotten and dispensable. The silence of the night brings you comfort as does the darkness outside. It's simple and predictable unlike the chaos within hospital walls. This simple silence can, however, be a double-edged sword. While it gives you space to breathe, it is also empty. You are all alone with your thoughts, and at times you feel cast away.

As the sun rises on a new day, society is rejuvenated and refreshed, yet you're exhausted. For the first time in your life you identify with the undesirable creatures lurking in the dark and pity them; for they are mostly misunderstood and nothing to be feared. A whole new dimension exists after dark and there's little insight into the vortex. You are expected to quietly and swiftly move in and out of the hospital without leaving a trace. Manage and keep the ship afloat regardless of the cost; keeping in mind there are no life vests available until day. Worried that if you shed a tear throughout the process you'll be labeled as dramatic or viewed as barbaric for passionately expressing yourself. But the truth is no one can function devoid of emotions. We cannot be well-oiled machines that simply continue to function regardless of the forces around us. There's a breaking point, even for the gentleman's monster.

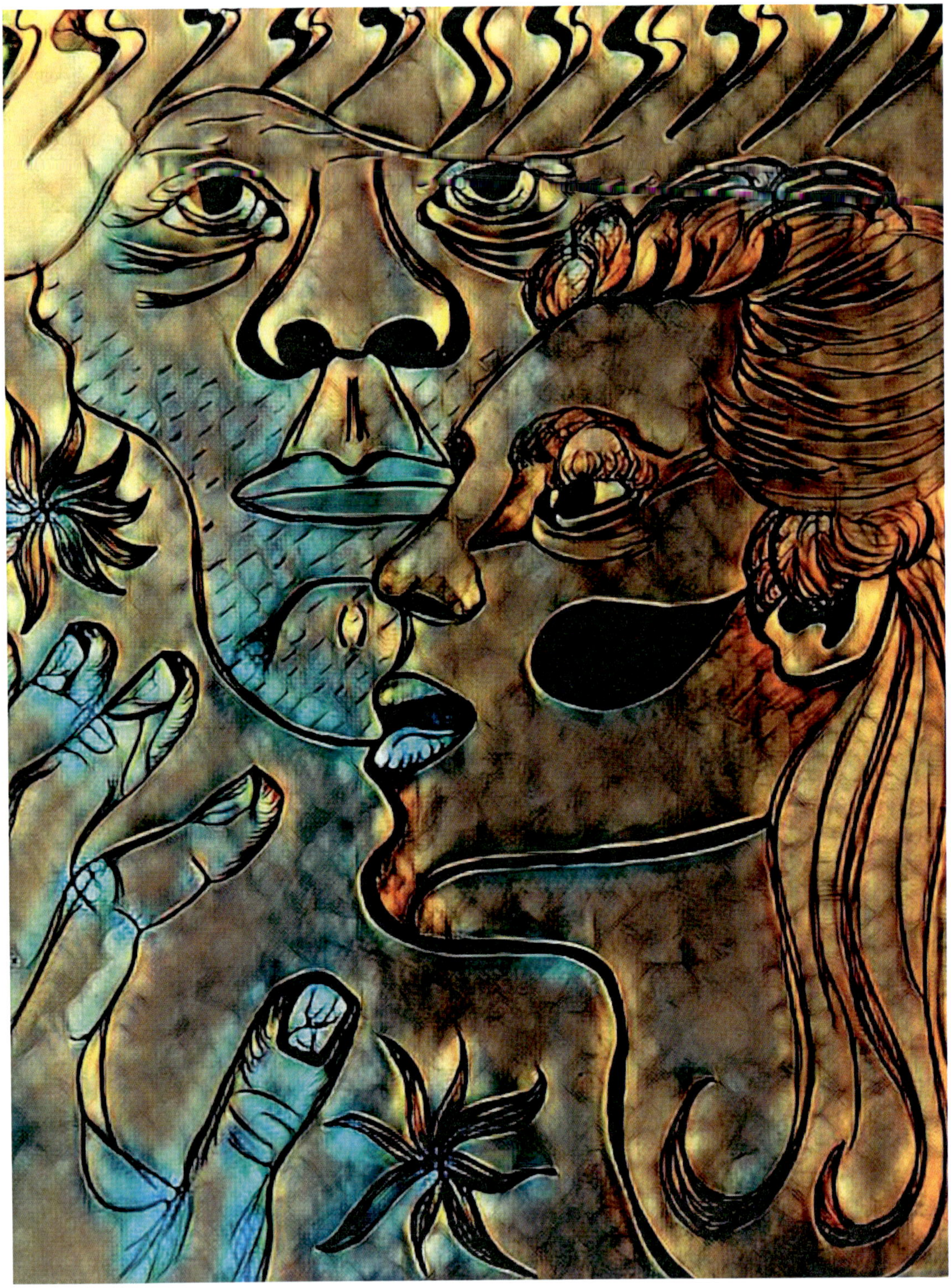

Chapter 5: Separation From Those We Love

Separation runs deep within the ICU and it can come in different forms. The physical, mental, and emotional toll of a patient's treatment and (hopefully) recovery at the level of intensive care is often extreme. Confusion, sedation, withdrawal from a substance, injury, and pain are all capable of drastically altering someone's persona. During this journey, those closest to the individual may feel as if their loved one is gone, even when that person is right in front of them. Further complicating this experience is the fact that most people who are critically ill do not look like themselves. There may be bandaging, bruising, swelling, tubes and machines seemingly fused to the body, etc...Unfortunately, many family and friends are left to wonder: will the person they knew ever come back? It's difficult because nurses often cannot provide answers to such questions, and we are all left relying only on time to tell.

Alone In The Dark

Invariably it's those moments when all is quiet and you're lying awake in the dark when you really start to miss someone; the lines on their face, their smell, the sound of their laugh. You start to imagine what it would be like to see them right here, right now. You'd give anything to have them. You'd even sell your soul to the devil himself for just a little more time. A restless mind leaves you wondering whether things would be like the good old days, or if maybe instead, you would be strangers now. It's a scary thought; to be unrecognizable to someone you love.

There are so many circumstances in life that can rip people apart, literally and figuratively. As nurses we see both routinely. It makes you want to run home and cover everyone you hold dear in bubble wrap. Is this extreme? Absolutely! However, the logic of wanting to protect the ones you love at all costs makes sense. Becoming fully aware that you lack control over what ultimately happens is simultaneously humbling and crippling. Ultimately, I think the thing that carries me through the fear is my belief that although love cannot prevent or fix everything, it can conquer all obstacles, even death. Whether this ideology is realistic or ignorant is something everyone must decide for themselves.

Wishful Longing

A hummingbird floats effortlessly from flower to flower with extreme precision through the most difficult conditions. His driving force is the need for fuel and energy that sustains him. The journey feeds his soul. So much so that he cannot stop. He craves it like a drug, and it consumes him.

All the while, a lotus bud lives deep beneath the water's surface. Surrounded by darkness for so long, she's grown tired. No longer does she feel this is what she deserves or where she belongs. Afraid to be seen, she blooms anyway and surges out of the shadows with a pure mind and heart.

Both are free spirits, one with wings and the other with roots; each bold and charming in their own way. Between the two there's enough fire and passion to set the world ablaze. Therefore, when the universe propels them together, the magic is unexplainable and unmistakable. But there's a problem. The hummingbird cannot stay, and the flower cannot go. Everyone knows what becomes of a flower plucked from the ground or a bird that cannot fly. So, with a heavy heart the hummingbird flies away. As the flower watches him leave, dewdrops fall from her petals, both spirits hoping and longing to be reunited someday.

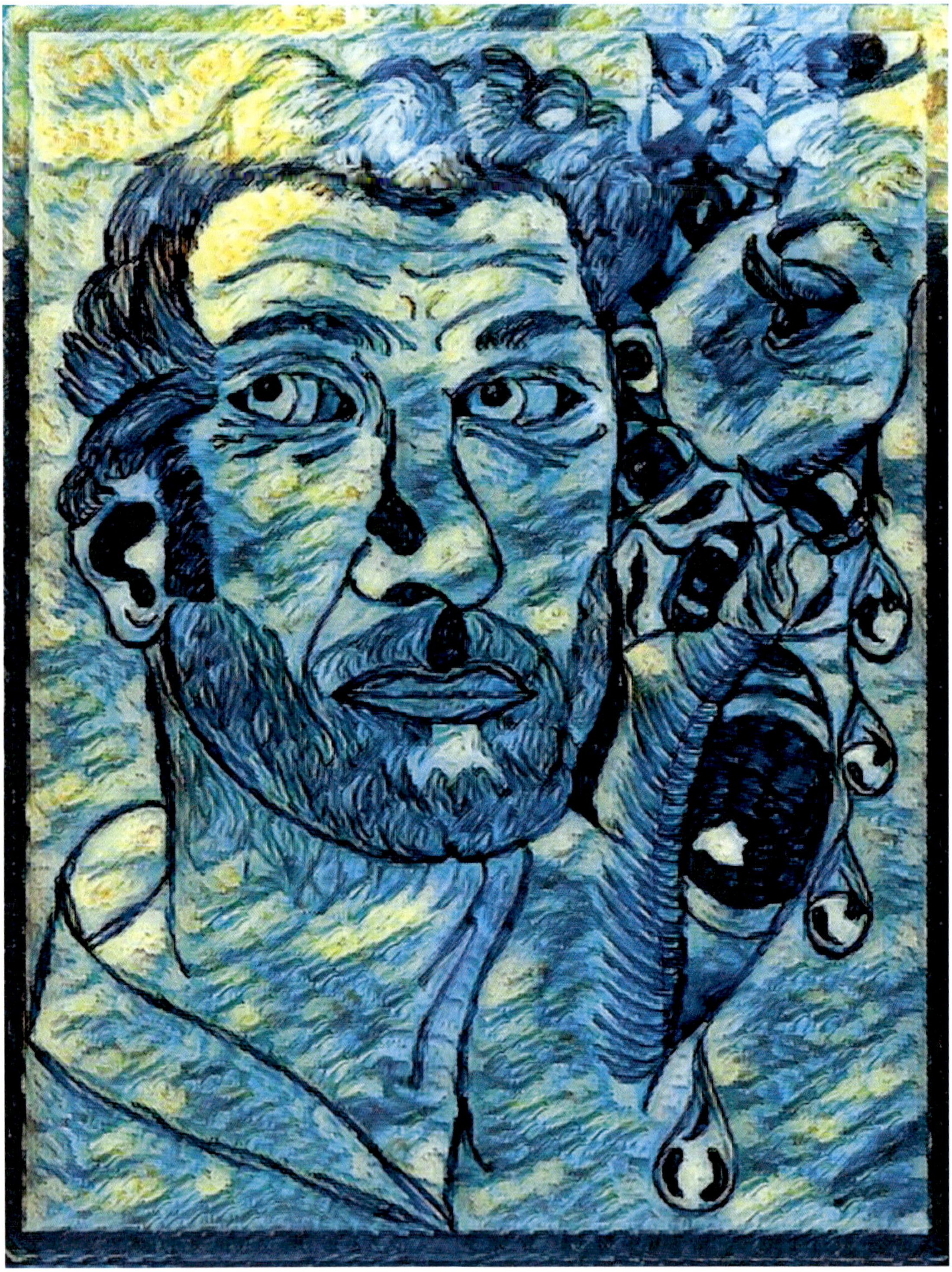

Chapter 6: Emotional Turmoil, Addiction, And Abuse

Emotional turmoil is tricky and frankly, it can be dangerous. We've all lost control of ourselves at some time or another. It's unnerving when our effective coping abilities seem to desert us, but stress and fear have a tendency to overtake our logical thought processes. What exactly triggers such a state is individually unique, as are the specifics of how each person ultimately deals with it. However, when emotional upheaval becomes extreme, damage to an individual's mental and/or physical wellbeing generally follows. In critical care, in order to heal someone, it's important to treat the damage done and also to find the source that triggered it.

Stop Running

The older I get, the more I appreciate time for reflection. Let's face it, life is busy, and we always seem to be spread too thin. Daily schedules are like a circus we've orchestrated for ourselves, one that we refuse to leave. We're eternally running, our minds and bodies in constant motion, which begs the question–what exactly are we running from?

Looking back on the much younger version of myself, I didn't realize that practicing self-love would be so difficult while keeping up with everything on my plate. But it seems that our perpetual busyness may be a symptom of seeking validation from others. Many people feel that they have something to prove by being constantly productive, perfectly groomed, highly successful, and always keeping a smile on their face while doing it. It's a dangerous game to play, especially if you forget to value yourself apart from all of that. It makes you dependent and subservient instead of free. I remember the first time I took myself to dinner, alone. I gave myself permission to slow down, take time for myself, and not care what others might think of a solo diner. It was the day I decided I was no longer broken, or at the very least, didn't want to be. Becoming comfortable in my own skin and choosing to be kind to myself, just as I am, are the greatest gifts I've given myself.

Within intensive care units we see a lack of self-love manifest itself in a variety of ways; depression, anxiety, substance abuse, self-harm, apathy, insomnia, harmful or dangerous sexual behaviors, rage, hopelessness, and on and on. Being a nurse, I get to see firsthand how many people need a little more love and kindness in their lives, especially from themselves.

Addiction

Addiction can be troublesome to understand and equally as difficult to treat. To be completely transparent, addicts are a gigantic segment of our patient population and are mentally taxing for the nurses taking care of them. Many of us unfortunately have experience with addiction in our personal lives whether it be a friend, a family member, or even we ourselves who struggle. Therefore, when we are presented with addiction at work, you can imagine how swiftly that hits a nerve on a very personal level. The physical and psychological effects of addiction are real, raw, and devastatingly obvious when you are a witness to someone hitting rock-bottom. Much of the time we never discover what leads people down this path and, regardless of the cause, it's heartbreaking. The worst part of it all is recognizing that some of these patients will be back, with their next hospital visit possibly being the last thing they do. It's an overwhelming internal struggle to realize that our job isn't to fix them. Instead, it's simply to be present and shed a little bit of light on them while they're in the dark.

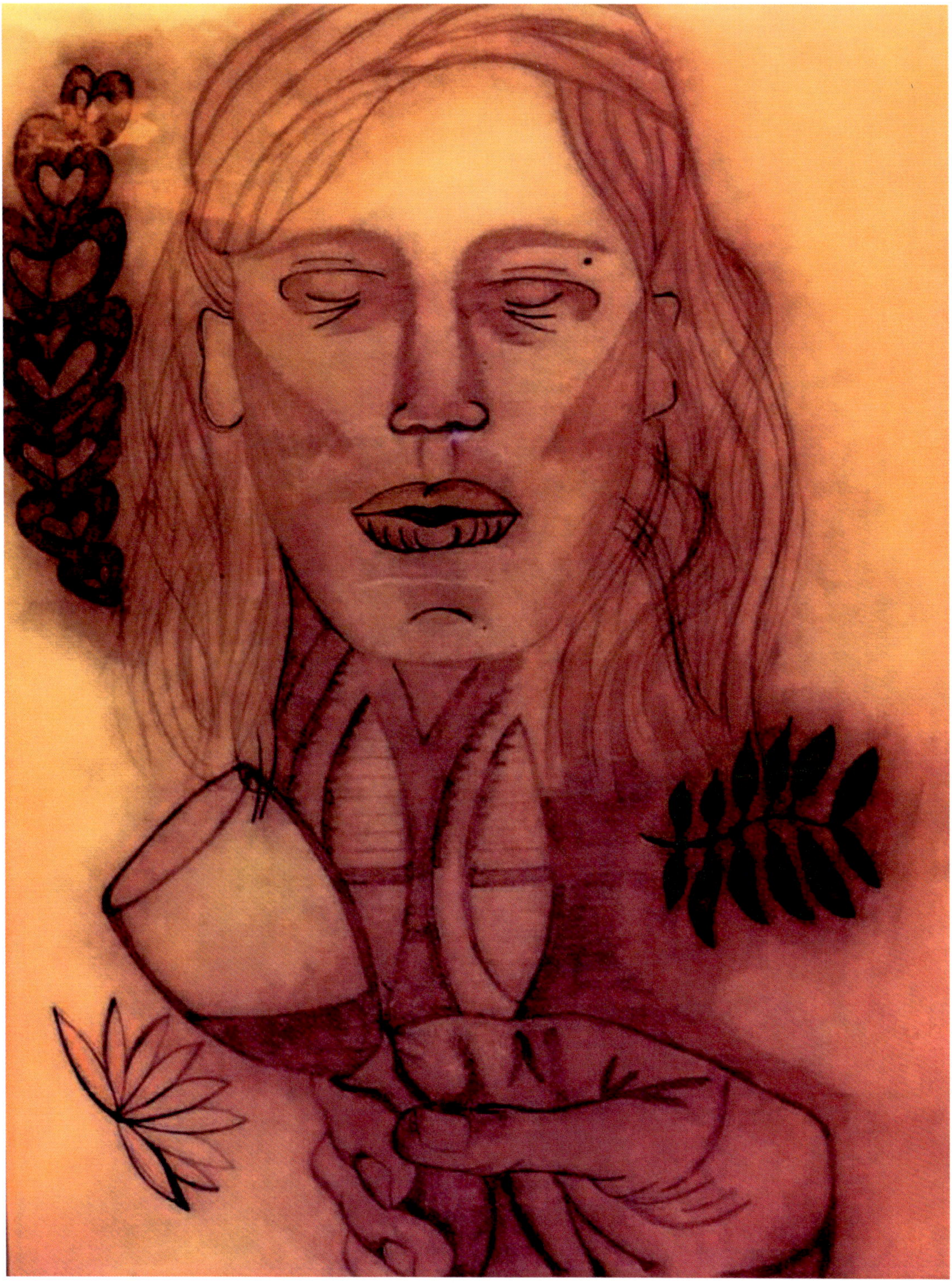

Is It Love Or Hate?

There's nothing quite like a good ol' lover's quarrel to get your blood pumping, literally. For centuries people have met their demise over romance, or lack thereof. You name it and we've seen it in intensive care. No one ever said love is painless.

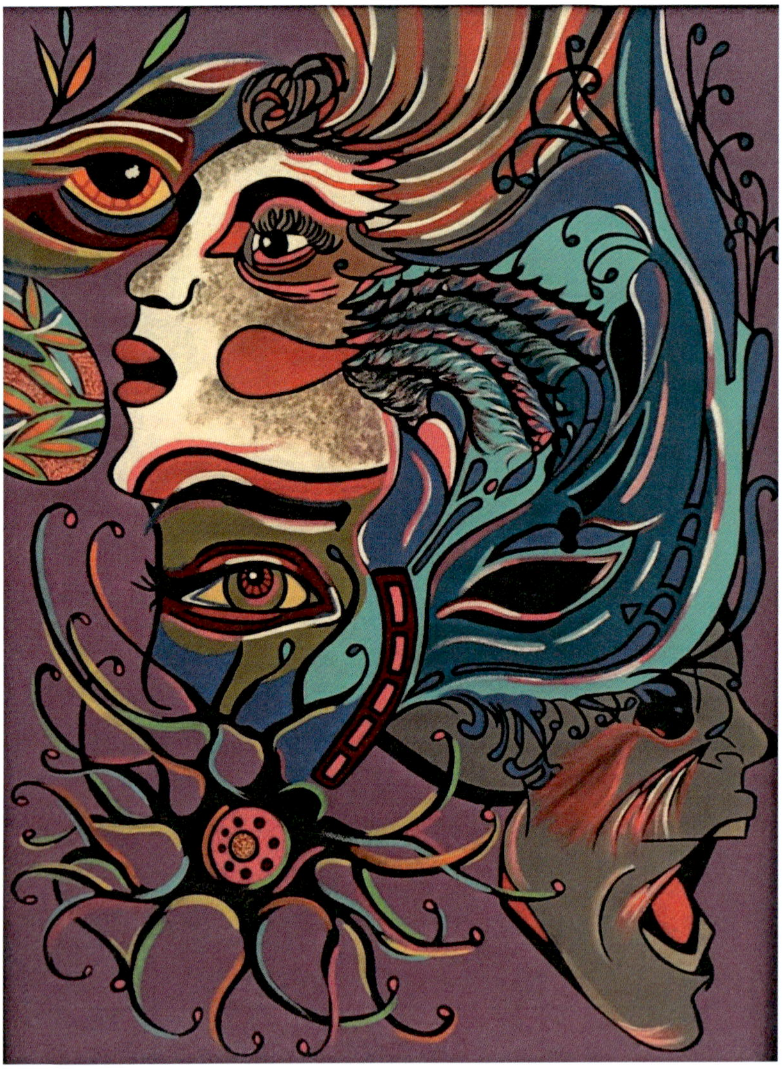

Abuse

Abuse affects us all. Whether we experience it ourselves or bear witness to its destructive force on someone else, the pain is real. So many burning questions loom around this topic. Many remain unanswered. As a nurse, when you are caring for a patient who has suffered at the hands of another, you cannot help but be angry. Hurting someone goes against everything you believe in and you wonder: if you looked upon the abuser, would you be looking pure evil in the face? You have a duty to protect your patients from harm. When confronted with cases of abuse, the need to protect only magnifies exponentially. Furthermore, there are a lot of nurses who have been in abusive relationships themselves. I've often thought that one of the reasons for this could be that nurses are such selfless creatures. I've also wondered if perhaps our dedication to fixing things may attract us to broken relationships. I don't know whether or not that is true, but I do know that these situations create complex emotions for all of us that we may never be able to fully process.

Utter Madness

Note: After speaking with so many individuals who have experienced abusive relationships or unhealthy affairs, I wanted to try to capture the dramatic effects such experiences have on one's psyche. This piece imagines a young woman who is attempting to understand her own emotional state in the immediate aftermath of such a relationship. It's important to note here that abuse happens to people of all ages, socioeconomic backgrounds, and to both genders. It's an epidemic that still needs our attention. This young woman, in particular, is desperate for answers. She feels as if she is going crazy. How could she possibly love someone who has hurt her so deeply? She seeks understanding not only of what happened, but also of herself.

I loved his madness. There's a flawed freedom that comes when you simply accept the utter confusion that overtakes your every breath. Not even my heart could reach him. Lost and wandering is where his soul remained, stuck inside a cage. Blind to the brutal truth, he fought for his prison rather than his release, while I listened intently to the lies he manufactured. I've always wondered what haunted him so deeply. Emotionally, he was locked in a safe without the code or key. When he finally flew away, he left behind a tangled mess. With wounds that run so deep in the aftermath, putting the pieces of the puzzle back together is complicated. Sadly, a piece of my heart will always belong to him. For what it's worth, I never want to ignore the truth, even if it's utter madness.

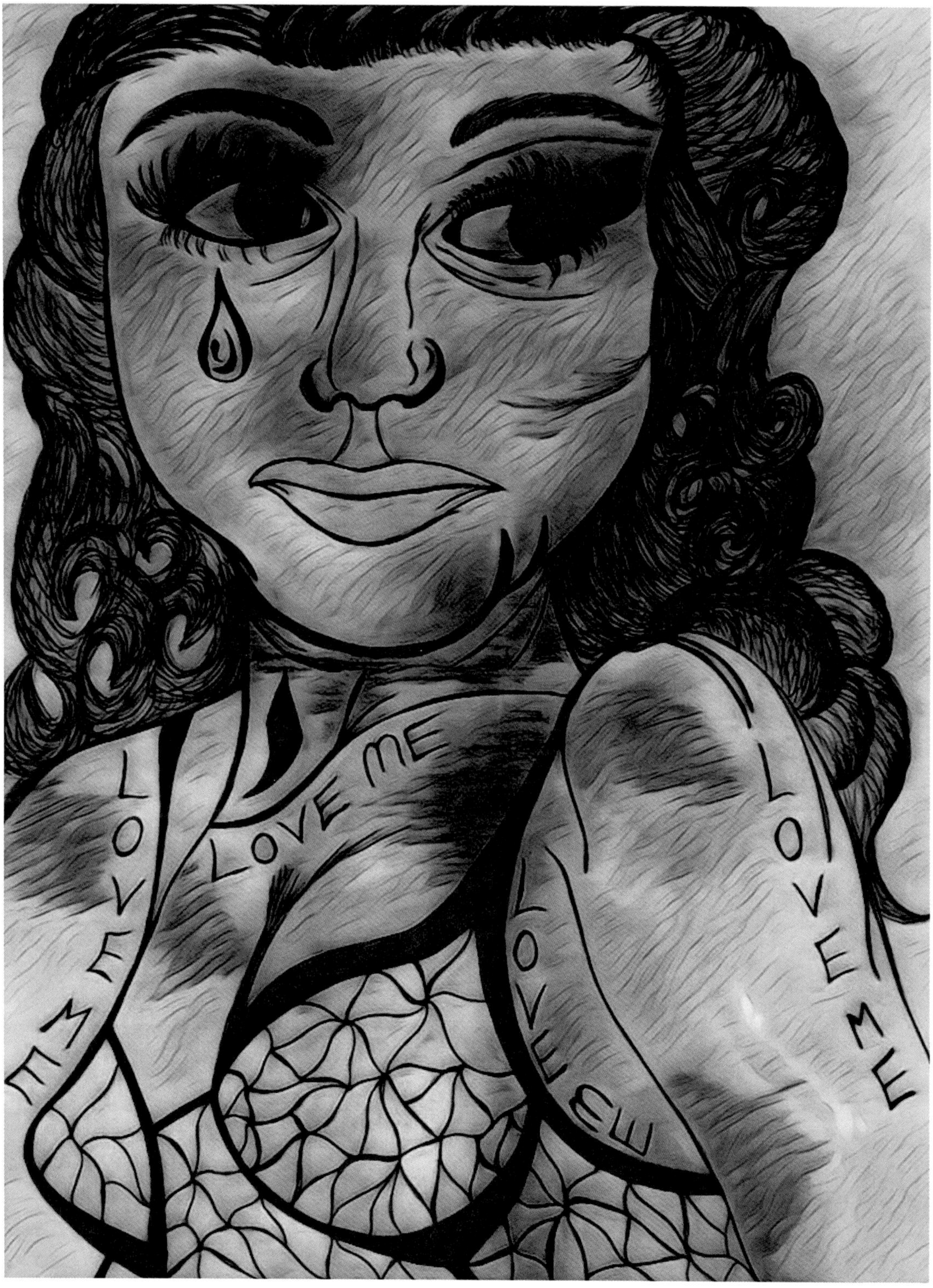
LOVE ME
LOVE ME
LOVE ME
LOVE ME

PTSD (Post-Traumatic Stress Disorder)

PTSD is still a grossly misunderstood phenomenon. Many of the patients in the ICU experience it simply because of the trauma of being horribly ill and tied to life-sustaining machines for prolonged periods of time. Other patients come in with the disorder as a result of previous trauma from abuse, war, or other violence. The level of fear and anxiety, and the ability to manage them varies from person to person, but the degree of compassion I feel for them is the same. Feeling as though your own body and mind are outside of your control must be haunting. The unpredictability of what might trigger an anxiety attack or cause a sleepless night would weigh heavily on anyone's heart. With so many uncertainties surrounding this disorder, the one thing I do know for sure is that these patients hold a special place in my own.

Note: The following poem is titled "The Beast", because I imagine that dealing with PTSD is much like fighting a beast. A patient once told me he felt as if he was fighting a battle with a mythical figure as well as himself. Another patient said she felt like the disorder was overtaking every part of her being. For these patients, PTSD affected everything from their quality of life, to their relationships and careers, slowly destroying everything. While everyone's journey with the disorder is different, the one commonality is that each individual wants their life back.

The Beast

For most people, sleep is easy.

It's effortless and peaceful.

A time for your mind and body to rest and rebuild,

but what if your mind never sleeps?

It takes two separate worlds and warps them into one,

and sometimes you cannot differentiate between a safe place and hell!

Your entire body is shaking, but you are not cold.

Drenched in sweat, your chest is heavy and it's hard to breathe.

Frantically, you sit hunched, searching for air,

clawing at the skin covering your body.

Hoping there's some form of protection still intact,

you scan the room for a ray of light amongst total darkness

and wait, alone, but the light never comes.

Your body begins to wilt

and your head falls down until it rests on your knees.

You tuck in your arms and hold yourself because no one is there to hold you,

but the beast is there patiently waiting.

He says he loves you.

He draws you in because he knows you're desperate.

In your mind you know he loathes you, but you give him pleasure.

So, he keeps you around

and punishes you for existing.

You convince yourself that if you pay your dues,

just maybe you can earn his respect.

Meanwhile, you pray for your prince;

a prince to rescue you.

Holding onto the notion that he exists,

your heart is overwhelmingly fragile.

You feel as if it might shatter with every beat.

You wonder if your prince will make it in time to save you,

because if he's too late,

you will either be dead at the hands of the beast,

or because of a broken heart!

Chapter 7: You Are Not Alone

I've been in that dark place where I've felt that I'd like to go to sleep, and just not wake up. It's a terrifying place to live. Sometimes you just want it all to stop. Everything and everyone has hurt you, and you've never felt so alone. No one could possibly understand; there's nothing to say that will take your pain away.

At one point, a very long time ago, I had a plan in place to make it all go away. At the time I felt that no one could possibly love a girl who was raped, beaten, and the owner of so many scars. Ultimately, my kids got me through because I realized that I didn't want to leave them. I didn't want them to feel alone the way I had. I've often wondered what my fate might have been had I not had them in my life. Honestly, it makes me shudder. I was so far down in the darkness that I almost didn't see the light again. Today, what I've come to understand is that I wasn't unlovable, but at that time I didn't love myself. It's taken me years to realize that my scars are powerful. They are my own personal map of my inner strength and the obstacles that I've overcome. I now wear them proudly and am able to openly discuss where I've been. Most importantly, I've learned that we all have something worth fighting for–that something is ourselves, because every life is worth living.

This chapter is about feeling alone and having a self-destructive ideology. Some people are fortunate because they are able to refocus and change the direction of their thoughts when they face difficulties in life. Others have been able to find some kind of a support system that gives them a lifeline.

However, there are those among us who find themselves unable to change course within their own minds when depression or trauma overtakes them. Unfortunately, their decisions in this state can have dire consequences mentally, physically, and spiritually.

Suicide

Suicide is a subject that captures our attention through shock. When this tragedy occurs, it inevitably takes us by surprise. Realistically, we can never have a complete picture of anyone's mental state. Each individual's thoughts are their own, which is both a blessing and a curse. We'd all like to think we are safe within our own minds, but that isn't always true for everyone. For some, thoughts lead down a path of misery and self-harm until life itself may seem too great a burden to bear.

Note: If you or someone you know is considering suicide please call:

The National Suicide Prevention Hotline

1-800-273-8255

(Support is available 24/7, free and confidential)

You are not alone!

The Edge: Choosing Life Or Death

In the midst of turmoil, you often find yourself searching for answers that will ease your heart and mind. However, processing trauma requires both willing participants to speak and perceptive listeners to hear. This is a combination that can be difficult to find. In your heart you are certain that you can be strong, but ironically, in order to become whole, you are forced to expose each and every weakness. Your mind and body have indulged themselves in a game of hide-and-seek. You want to lose that which must be found. A battle rages between acknowledgement and denial. You stand perched on the edge, but not because you are waiting to fall and not because you are looking for someone to catch you. Instead, you are wondering if anyone will even notice.

See the note on p. 69 for the National Suicide Hotline

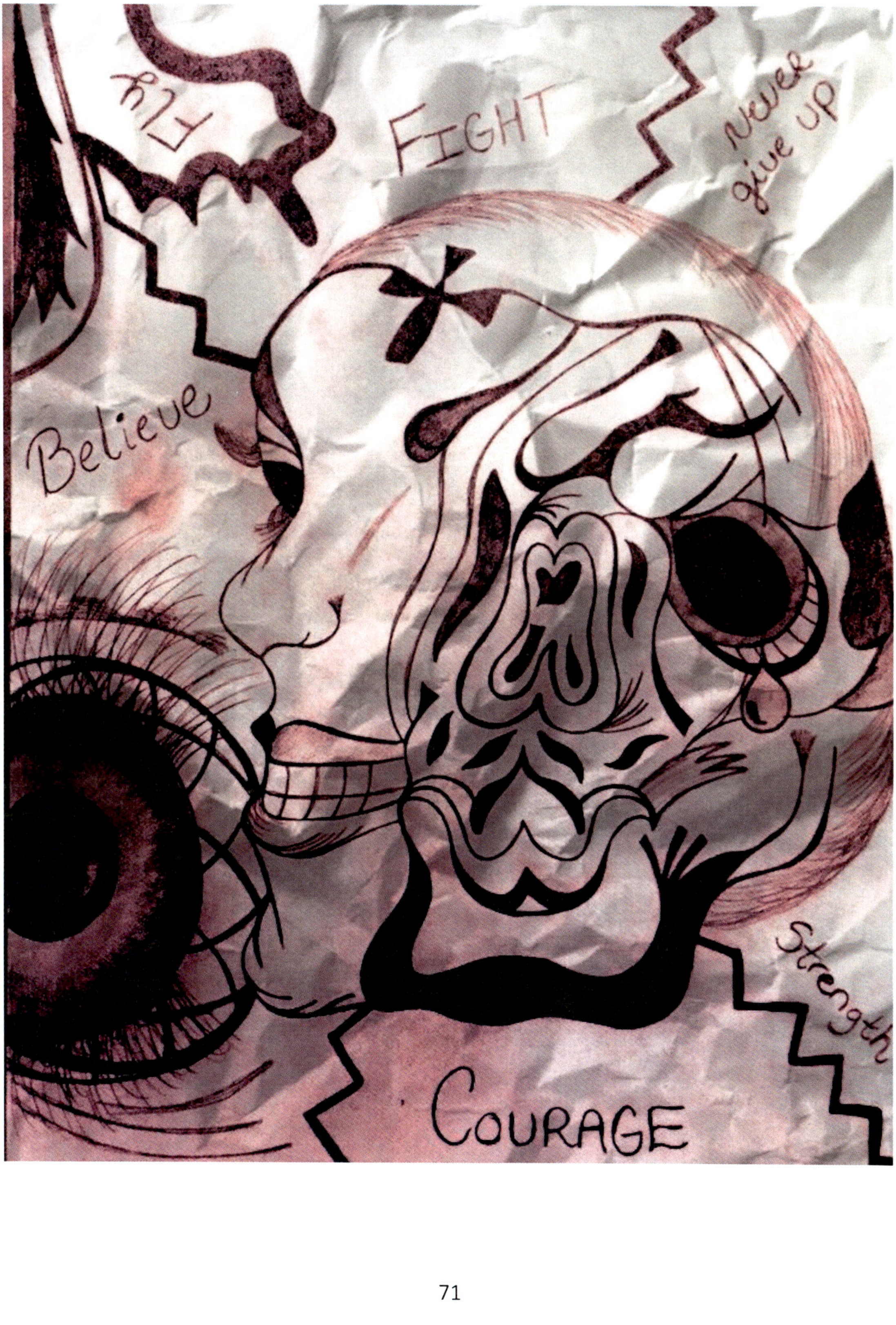
Fly
FIGHT
Never give up
Believe
Strength
COURAGE

Loneliness

Within the ICU, I've been a witness to so much loneliness. While most of us spend much of our lives surrounded by other people, feeling connected to a community can be a significant challenge. Being an independent person myself, I often embrace solitude. Just ask anyone who knows me! I'm not afraid to treat myself to a solo dinner out or an occasional glass of wine at the bar all by myself. That being said, I always feel supported by my friends and family. I know they are there for me when I need them. Unfortunately, a lot of people don't have that support network. Many are uncomfortable reaching out or phoning someone for help, while some simply don't have anyone at all that they can reach out to. As a result, they end up in my unit due to a lack of mental, physical, and/or social support systems. I understand that needing critical care because of loneliness could seem like a very nebulous concept. However, when people feel alone, they often forget to take care of themselves or they feel unable to access resources to improve an unsustainable living situation. As a result, they may become injured or their health deteriorates to an alarming state.

I'm not sure how to fix this problem, but I definitely believe in my heart that loneliness is an epidemic. Creating meaningful human connection in this day and age requires intentionality. It requires us to take notice of opportunities to reach out to those around us, even in very small ways. So for now, my goal is to always change someone's day for the better. Sometimes that means something as simple as smiling at someone when I catch their eye, or paying for a stranger's coffee. You never know, you might save someone's life with kindness.

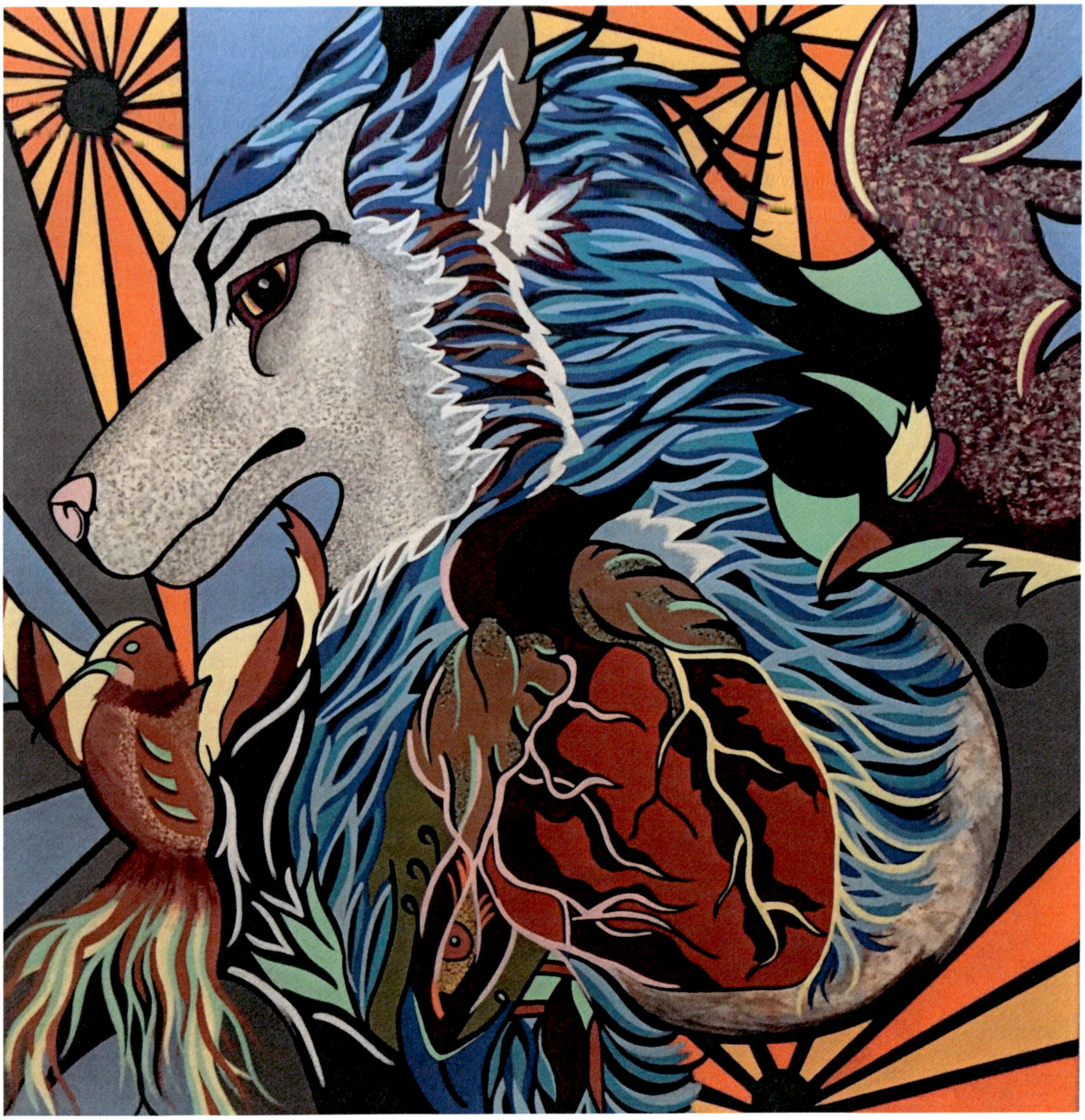

The Statue

There is an alluring statue watching over everyone.
One glance and his face tells a story,
he is stoic but weary with burdens.
Who watches over him?
Handsome yet vulnerable,
his emotions transcend the outer shell he has created.
Appearing unbreakable and unphased by all external elements;
his soul longs for warmth,
but who could love this statue?
There are days where he gathers up the courage,
opens his heart and reaches out his hand.
He chants over and over!
With his eyes closed, he prays for someone to be there,
but upon opening his eyes he finds himself alone in the rain;
with nothing but hope to hold onto.

Self-Loathing

Masquerade balls are something of a personal fascination for me. Celebrations where people hide their true selves are both captivating and curious. We as a society have conditioned ourselves to embrace "masks". In fact, we look forward to parties and events that allow us to embody different characters by dressing up in costumes. Over time, I've wondered if this obsession is the result of people being uncomfortable in their own skin. Working in a profession where I interact with large volumes of people every day, I am a direct witness to the concept that other people's perceptions rule our lives. It's saddening because rather than searching for ways in which we can be better versions of ourselves, many of us are actually trying to *be* someone else. As a result, we attempt to mold our personalities and physical appearances into forms that are considered more desirable by society. In effect, we are donning "masks" to present to the world.

In addition to creating streamlined images for ourselves, we strive for more money, more possessions, or better relationships in hopes of finding happiness. We are working to keep up appearances so that we can meet the expectations we imagine others have of us, while satisfying our own distorted images of perfection. Through it all, the hard truth is that happiness doesn't live there. Instead, it lives in acceptance of who we are, imperfections and all. We may not really be wearing masks in public, but we certainly aren't advertising our true selves. So, take off the "mask" my love, because the real you is beautiful.

Note: The next poem is about a figurative mask that rules an individual's life. Being authentic is something so many people struggle with. Dependence on a fake persona becomes necessary for survival. Trying to break away from personal and societal expectations can make us feel exposed. My hope is that we all find it in our hearts to foster acceptance and love for differences, so that no one feels they have to wear a mask ever again.

The Mask

Tears of heartache, tears of pain,
a raging river locked away, not meant to be contained.
Behind a mask,
but the mask is not me.
I still scream.
I suffer in silence behind this mask I made.
As much as I hate my mask, it comforts me,
because I cannot see or feel my pain.
It shields me, protects me.
Feeling nothing is better than feeling everything,
or is it?
To feel nothing is the same as to disappear, to be insignificant,
but there is too much pain,
too much sadness,
too much heartache,
from the past and present.
It still comes for me.
It's the demon waiting patiently for day to turn to night;
the phantom who longs for its prey to be alone.
It smiles because it senses my fear, the fear that keeps me imprisoned.
Forced to conform and sworn to silence, I try to cover my scars.

I reach for my mask, but I cannot hide.

Helpless, I pray, but there is no answer.

When it is over, I sit exposed, relieved and overwhelmed.

I lock away my tears; breathe to know I am alive,

and I reach for my mask.

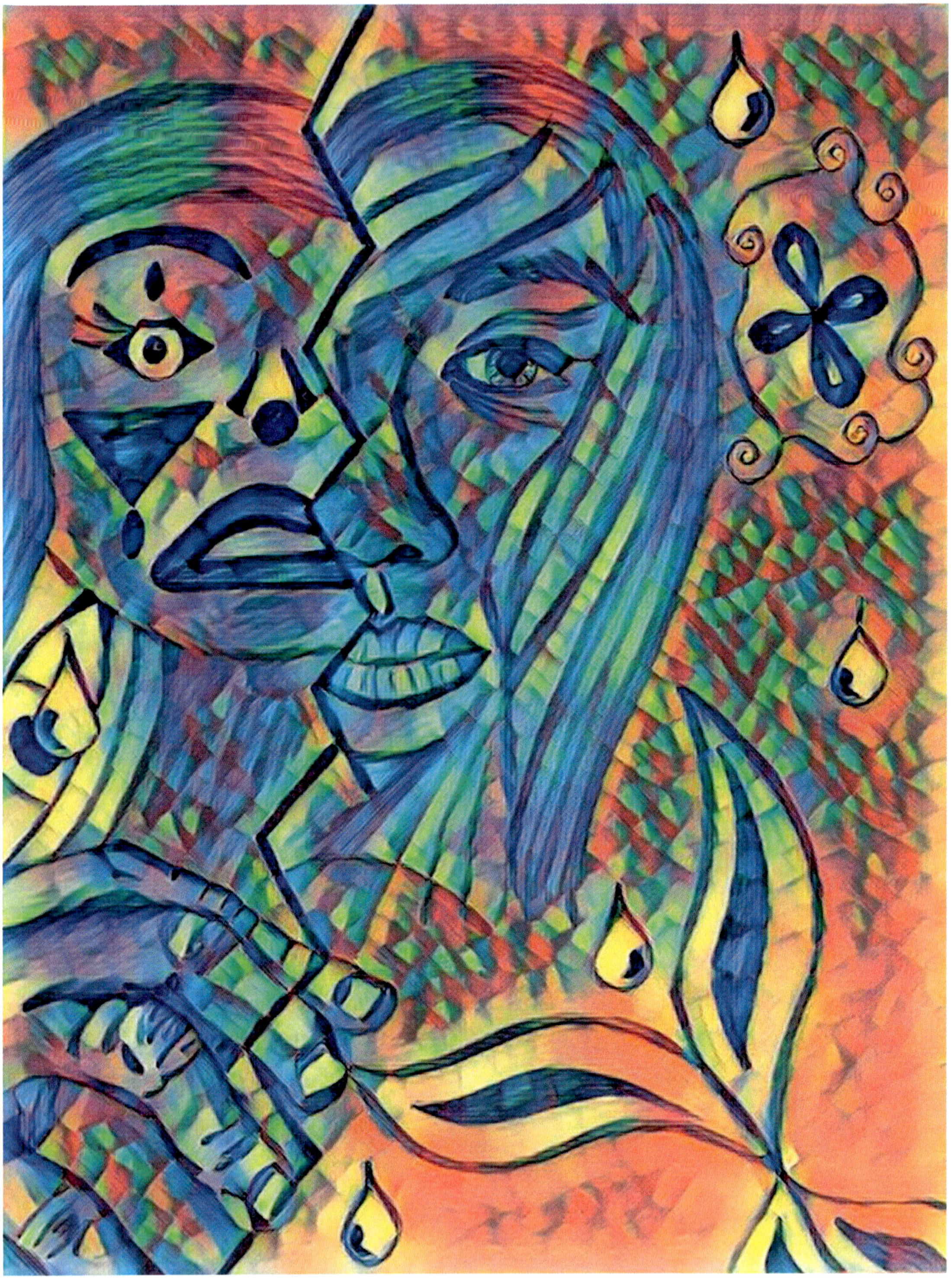

Chapter 8: The Soul Of A Nurse

Being a nurse is not just a job. It's a duty and a promise you make to all mankind, as well as to yourself. You're dedicating your life to a purpose and a passion. It's a lifelong commitment in a world that doesn't seem to value such consistency. Since the beginning of time, there have always been individuals who were naturally drawn to healing others. Making sick people well again was their obsession. Many were called witches and wizards; they were persecuted and even sentenced to death for propelling science over the priest. Let's be clear, there's no reason we cannot believe in both, but that fact was not always accepted. During certain times in our history, the "magical powers" of healers were feared. Fortunately, the prospect of attracting suspicion, enduring torture, and even threats of death have all failed to deter the pursuit of medical knowledge. Such conviction in our purpose could be the most breathtaking aspect of nursing and the medical profession overall. The willingness to surrender oneself to such a purpose offers a glimpse into the soul of a nurse.

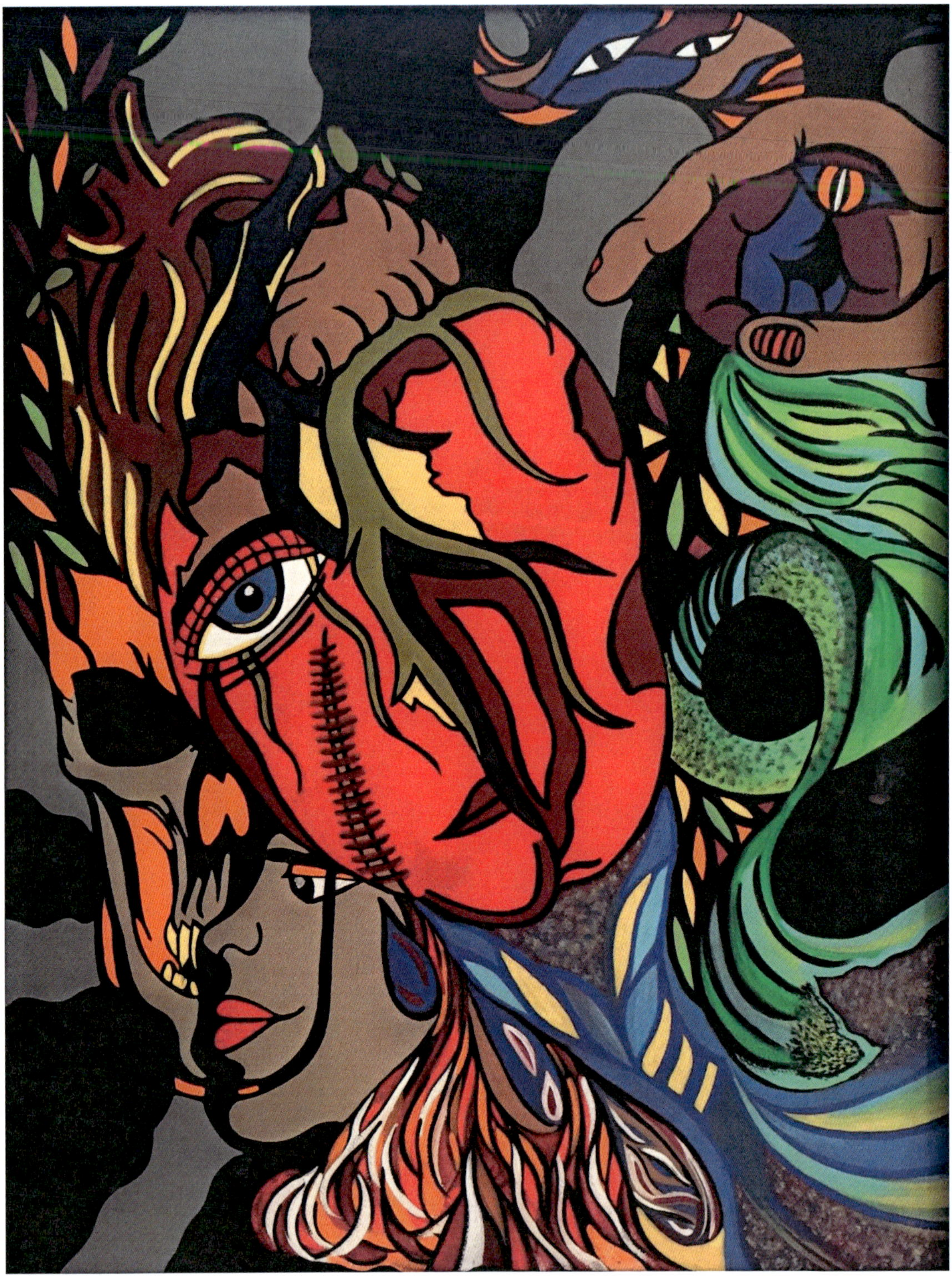

The Little Things

It's incredible how much I value the little things now. After working in an environment where I'm constantly surrounded by extreme situations and frequently witness insurmountable illness, I have a heightened appreciation for normal daily rituals and small pleasures. Things like my morning coffee, driving around town, or a stunning sunset just seem to hold so much more significance than they once did. Everything you've ever known could be stripped away in an instant, but most of us take our lives for granted. We become wrapped up in the daily grind and simply forget to enjoy what we have.

One of my favorite things to do is go out, find a cozy spot, and people-watch. I like to see people living their lives, laughing, sharing happy moments with family or friends. Those little snapshots are so refreshing because a huge portion of my own life is spent witnessing the other side of things–pain, fear, and loss. I've perfected the art of being a support for others in their time of need, and I do love being there for them. The challenge is not getting lost or stuck in that emotional space, which is easier said than done. There's always a tipping point for every nurse where they become cognizant of the fact that they are taking their work home with them. The challenge then becomes being able to set all of that aside, at the proper time, to make space for joy in your life.

The Blue Rose

The other day I was walking through a farmer's market, picking out an arrangement of roses, and I started thinking about the power of choice. The world we live in is colored by our decisions every day. We build our surroundings in a similar fashion to the way we build a bouquet. We design, customize, and choose to integrate what ultimately speaks to us. Throughout my life, I've always been drawn to blue roses and until this day in the marketplace, I never knew the meaning behind them. The vendor, who I could sense was a spiritual man, leaned over and asked me if I was a healer. At first, I was a little taken aback; how could he possibly know I'm a nurse? It turns out that he'd seen me there before and I always bought blue roses. He told me that they are symbols of protection and strength. He had always wondered whether I needed protection or if, in fact, I protected others in some way.

On this day I was standing with my blue roses next to a rock I'd never noticed before. Painted on it was a symbol known as the Healer's Hand. The vender explained to me that my energy, the roses, and my standing next to this symbol led him to believe that I had to be some kind of a healer. It was one of the most intriguing conversations of my life. We had never formally met yet he knew so much about me.

During our conversation he told me that some flowers are colored by nature and others, like the blue roses, must be colored by the grower. He emphasized that we can learn so much about ourselves through flowers. To me this was a beautiful comparison that I had never even considered. “If we desire something to be, we have the power to make those desires come true, just as I've made this rose a beautiful blue”, he said, “but there are some things we cannot change, for this flower is also beautiful simply for what it is all by itself–a rose.” He kissed me on the cheek and whispered, “Be well my child. You have a compassionate heart. Keep spreading love and people will see your soul.” And then, he disappeared. It was almost as if he magically vanished and I suddenly stood alone, surrounded by flowers. To this day I still wonder if I had this encounter because I had been doubting myself and my own choices. Maybe having gone through my own struggles and acquiring some scars, I needed to hear that I was still beautiful. Or maybe, I needed reassurance that I held the power to decorate my own world with the bouquet of my choice. I don't think I will ever have the answers to these burning questions and maybe that's the point. What I do know is that a blue rose, to me, is now so much more than a flower.

For The Love Of Critical Care

Critical care is one of the loves of my life. I've never been a part of anything else that has required me to open my heart so freely and also to think so eloquently. The head and the heart don't always work together because love is blind, and being led by one's heart frequently means forgoing rational thought. In this instance however, they are the perfect pairing. The ICU is a place where passion for people and pathophysiology (the physical manifestation of illness or injury) are necessary for success. In critical care you get to be both a lover and a fighter, and I find that I feel at home within that paradox. While life can seem to require you to choose between a logical mind and a passionate heart, the beauty of critical care is that it never requires that choice.

Walking The Line

For ICU nurses, the sound of a ventilator, the rhythmic beats echoing from a telemonitor, or the continuous churning noises of a dialysis machine can be comforting. We are accustomed to these sounds that indicate we are where we belong, doing work that is vitally important. When we nurses are caring for our patients, we are in our element. The familiarity of this environment is soothing because, similar to the development of muscle memory, our brains know exactly what to do and how to do it from rigorous training and practice.

I've never been as confident in myself or in my abilities as I am while taking care of someone who is critically ill. This may seem odd because critical care is defined by uncertainty. The very nature of the conditions for which a patient is placed in the intensive care unit means that situations can turn on a dime and outcomes are not always clear. But despite the cards at play, I know my years of training will take over when the need arises. Time seems to stand still when someone teeters on the boundary between life and death. I become immersed in a dance, effortlessly flowing. The music playing in my head is about the disordered physiologic processes occurring and how to correct them. It is a foreign universe, an alternate dimension that not many people enter; I welcome it, because fighting for a life is something that I'll eternally walk the line for.

Chapter 9: Beautiful Endings

This last chapter is about endings. All things must come to an end, including, of course, life. Throughout all the years I've been an ICU nurse, endings have been an ever-present part of my life's work. At first, I didn't know how to deal with that and I felt lost, but now I see things more clearly. I see the hope and beauty in uncertainty *and* in finality. When I entered the nursing profession, I wanted to make a difference in the lives of others. I had no idea that on this journey, I'd actually find myself immensely and very personally impacted by those I am caring for. Through it all, I've learned to take notice of what is beautiful in myself and in my surroundings. Even more importantly, I've learned that though there will always be endings, often accompanied by sadness, there will also be new beginnings. There is beauty, peace, and hope in recognizing the blessings of both.

Adoration

Critical care gives us a beautiful ending to many true love stories. I can't even tell you how much I cherish listening to people talk about how they met their partners and about their lives together. It makes you believe again in things like fairy tales and love at first sight; you can regain a bit of the childlike innocence you tend to lose as an adult. I once spoke with a gentleman about his lovely wife during her final hours. His devotion to her was obvious. My only hope is that everyone finds a fraction of the love that couple shared.

The following essay, My Phoenix (p. 90), is a snapshot of this couple's love story. It is only written from the gentleman's perspective because I never had the opportunity to speak with his wife. I feel fortunate to have heard him speak of all the qualities he loved about her. When writing this piece there were so many areas in which I wanted to take creative liberties and fill in the gaps about this love story, but I couldn't bring myself to do it. I have left the text in the form in which it was related to me and therefore, it is open to the interpretation of the reader. Instead of reading a story that makes perfect sense, we are being allowed a small glimpse into this gentleman's heart.

My Phoenix

She was completely confusing. Her spirit did not belong to anyone or anything, but rather a mission which was to be unapologetically herself. She was a rebel with a cause who wanted to spread love in a world consumed by judgement and hate. Back when we were young, getting married and starting a family was expected. Women were courted constantly, and this made her feel like she was a route to be conquered. You see, she refused to be seen as some man's expedition. Instead, she sought adventure and loved her life all by herself. She was the opposite of cliché, and it was possibly her most intriguing quality. She vowed to care for everyone, even those others might find undeserving; so many believed her to be crazy because of it.

Oddly enough, she never minded being misunderstood; she welcomed the critics. Controversy builds character and creating change seldom comes without controversy. Her silent strength made a statement louder than words. Many questioned her life choices because of her passion for travel; she had an intense desire for the unknown. These decisions made her quite unpopular amongst her peers. Even though others laughed at her for what they interpreted as mental instability, she never felt the need to be outspoken, as final words are for fools and a mockery she was not.

A flower and a Phoenix are how I came to see her because both are representations of new life, and she completely changed mine. She gave her heart to all, but never sacrificed her soul for anyone or anything, and I loved her for it.

Hope

Through all the experiences I've had as a nurse, there's one consistent message: hope. There is always hope. It is present in the patients and families we care for, and it is present in us as well. Without it, there's no way we could move forward through life's ever-present trials and tribulations. In my opinion, hope is the most sacred state of mind and should be protected as well as cherished. Now, exactly how we do so is where creativity and individuality take over. Most importantly, hope is not necessarily the promise of things working out in your favor; it's much deeper and more complex.

I've seen so many cases where people have hoped for strength, for peace, or simply for the desire to smile once again. I truly believe that hope represents all of these desires and so many more that are fluid and ever-changing, rather than static. Hope keeps people moving forward. We certainly cannot predict the future, but we can encourage people to keep their spirits alive; we can let them know that we are listening and that we are hoping with them. With that in mind, as this book comes to a close, it seems appropriate to end with this message:

Even in your darkest hour, hope and love are with you always!

To My Readers

A special thank you to all my readers! Your support for this project will help promote mental health amongst those in the nursing profession. In doing so, hopefully we can create a culture that revolves around us taking care of each other just as much as we take care of our patients. Lastly, thank you to all the nurses out there for doing what you do every day!

Dedication

This book is dedicated to the wonderful nursing community I am so blessed to be a part of and the team of exceptional nurses I have the privilege of working with on a daily basis. To all my friends and family, for your overwhelming support on this project, thank you. Last, but not least, a special shout out to my mother, my father in heaven, my brother, and my kids for always being there for me. I love you more than words can express!

Pages For Your Thoughts

I've Included extra pages here at the end of this book to encourage my readers to express themselves and create healthy outlets for whatever battles they may be fighting.

Pages For Your Thoughts

Grab a coffee after work, phone a friend, or even sit in the car for a cry session. Your emotions are meaningful and valid. Don't ignore them!

Pages For Your Thoughts

What have you done to take care of yourself today?

Pages For Your Thoughts

Love yourself!

Pages For Your Thoughts

Life is all about balance; don't lose yours!

YOU ARE....

BEAUTIFUL

STRONG

POWERFUL

IMPACTFUL

COMPASSIONATE

LOVED

REMEMBER TO....

HAVE COURAGE
FIND STRENGTH
BELIEVE
AND
LOVE

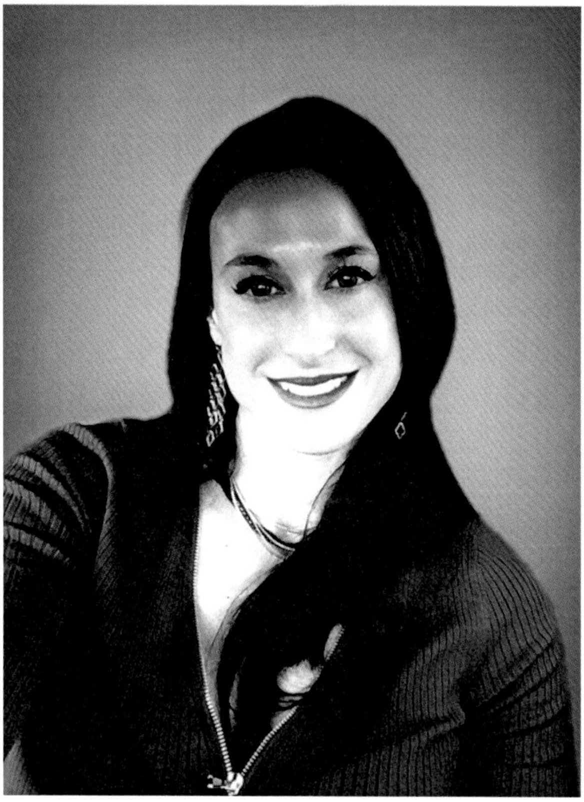

About the Author

Pamela Karakusis has been an ICU (Intensive Care Unit) nurse at a level one trauma center for the entirety of her career. Over the years, in dealing with high-acuity assignments and complex patient processes, she realized that a focus on mental health for nurses was lacking. In an effort to help herself deal with the daily difficulties of her job, she started a journal that included her own written and artistic expressions about her experiences. Pamela was recently recognized by the Daisy Foundation for exceptional and compassionate nursing care. She was also recognized as a leader in her field when she was published in the 2018 edition of *Worldwide Leaders in Healthcare*. Currently, Pamela is working as a Clinical Nurse Coordinator in a trauma ICU. Her mission and passion in life continues to be helping others.

Made in United States
North Haven, CT
05 November 2026

21763977R60062